ENJOY THE MOST FLAVORFUL
RECIPES UNDER THE SUN.

THE SONOMA DIET™ Cookbook

DR. CONNIE GUTTERSEN, R.D., PH.D.

Meredith® Books • Des Moines, Iowa

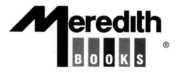

Meredith Books
1716 Locust Street
Des Moines, Iowa 50309–3023
www.meredithbooks.com

First Edition.
Printed in the United States of America.
Library of Congress Control Number: 2006921324
ISBN-13: 978-0-696-23185-8
ISBN-10: 0-696-23185-9

Table of Contents

Acknowledgments

Northern California's wine country, known for rolling hills of vines, bountiful fruits and vegetables, and incredible seafood from the Pacific, has inspired me to bring together the pleasures of the table with a healthy lifestyle. It also provides a model for those who seek weight loss as part of an easy-to-follow plan with flavorful foods.

I appreciate the tremendous motivation my late father, Bruno Peraglie, M.D., instilled in me to explore the science of food and nutrition for attaining better health. It's an idea that comes to life today as we understand how foods and lifestyle can improve health and prevent the many diseases that afflict us. With sincere gratitude, I would also like to thank my mother, Paola Peraglie, who provided me with a lifetime of lessons on how to enjoy and prepare delicious meals. Her philosophy of simple preparations using natural foods and a touch of creativity are woven into these recipes.

Thank you to Chef Toni Sakaguchi and the late Chef Catherine Brandel for their culinary inspiration. They introduced me to taste experiences that now are at the cornerstone of my philosophy that flavorful foods are key to the success of a healthy lifestyle and way of eating. I would like to also acknowledge The Culinary Institute of America at Greystone for the opportunity to learn about the exciting flavors that await us throughout the world. Incorporating these world flavors as part of a plan to teach America how to eat healthy remains an incredible endeavor for me to fulfill.

My appreciation and gratitude to The Sonoma Diet team for their knowledge, time, and effort: Jim Blume, Doug Guendel, Bob Mate, Patrick Taylor, Jennifer Darling, Stephanie Karpinske, Kelly Garrett, Amy Nichols, Gina Rickert, Jennifer Vogel, Steve Rogers, Greg Kayko, Ken Zagor, Margie Schenkelberg, Matt Strelecki, Som Inthalangsy, Andy Lyons, and Laura Harms. A special thank you to Heidi Krupp and her incredible Krupp team for their tremendous enthusiasm and expertise.

I would like to thank my husband, Shawn, and children, Gabriella and William, for their support and enthusiasm for my endeavors in teaching nutrition and The Sonoma Diet.

{ FROM THE AUTHOR }

Welcome to *The Sonoma Diet Cookbook*, the greatly anticipated companion to *The Sonoma Diet* book. Inspired by the Mediterranean way of eating and touched by the global flavors of Asia and Latin America, The Sonoma Diet makes it easy to lose weight and gain health with delicious and satisfying foods. *The Sonoma Diet Cookbook* brings you even more delicious recipes to keep you living this satisfying, new way of eating. You'll find recipes bursting with flavor yet still true to the principles of this successful weight loss plan. Each bite captures the essence of California wine country cuisine.

Working with chefs at The Culinary Institute of America has taught me that great-tasting food can be healthy and easy to prepare. You just need to know how to bring out the many unique and wonderful flavors in food. In this book, I've included some simple ways to do just that—using aromatic herbs and spices combined with healthful, wholesome foods. Whether it's a Moroccan spice rub or an Asian herb rub you add to your favorite meat, you'll find that a little seasoning makes a big difference in even the most basic foods.

This cookbook may say "diet" on the cover, but it's much more than that. It invites you to explore the endless possibilities of food combinations that bring the wine country's sun-drenched flavors to your home. Enjoy this collection of recipes with your entire family as part of a healthier lifestyle. And live life to the fullest with great, flavorful food.

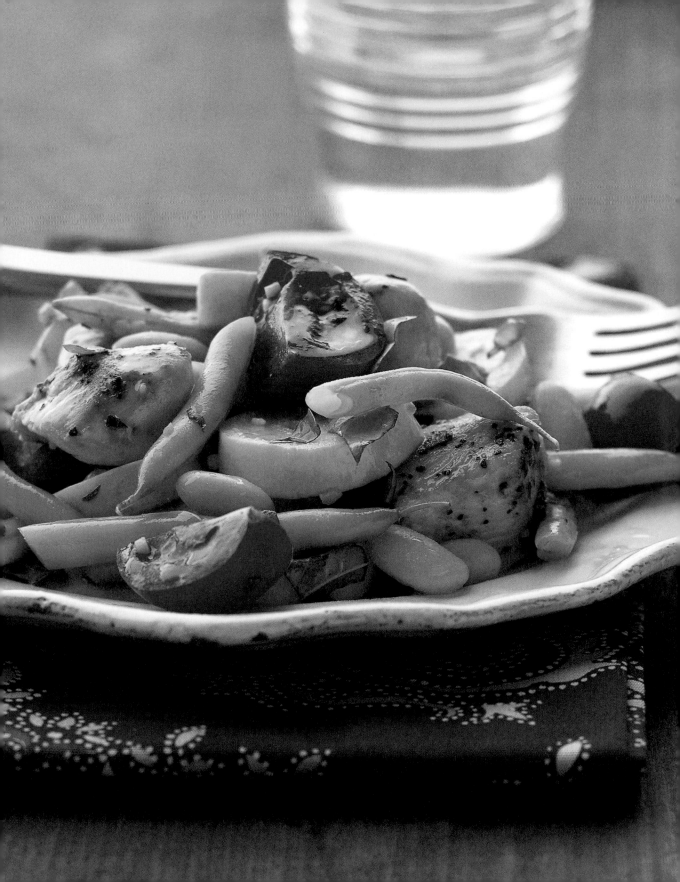

Flavor in Every Bite

The remarkable success of *The Sonoma Diet* is
based on a simple idea: The surest route to healthy
weight loss is to enjoy delicious, wholesome foods
in satisfying amounts every day. Many people have
already tried this healthy way of eating and have
experienced the exciting results.

Knowing how good it feels to savor the flavorful,
healthy meals of The Sonoma Diet, it's only
natural to want to explore more of these tastes
from the Mediterranean, Asia, and Latin America.
The Sonoma Diet Cookbook exists for just that
purpose. In the pages, you'll find more than
200 mouthwatering recipes, all inspired by the
sundrenched landscapes and fertile soils of the diet's
birthplace—California's Sonoma County. You'll also
find lots of ideas to ensure the variety and fresh
mealtime pleasure that are so essential to your
new Sonoma Diet lifestyle.

Flip through these recipes and you'll be enticed by the simplicity and delicious flavor profiles. The foods are far beyond what many have come to expect from "diet" foods. But every one of the recipes has been designed to fit right into your Sonoma Diet, no matter how far along you are. If you're just starting on the diet, you'll find plenty of options for Wave 1, which is a 10-day period to jump-start your weight loss. Those on Wave 2 will find the variety and adventure they need to get the most out of this longer-term, steady weight loss phase of the diet.

And those on Wave 3, the ones looking to take advantage of the Sonoma Diet lifestyle for years after they've reached their target weight? There's enough information and inspiration in these pages to keep you fit for a lifetime.

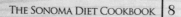

Enjoy Wholesome Foods

The Sonoma Diet is synonymous with pure and delicious, wholesome foods. At the core of this are the 10 Sonoma Diet Power Foods: extra-virgin olive oil, almonds, bell peppers, broccoli, tomatoes, spinach, grapes, strawberries, blueberries, and whole grains. These foods help you lose weight and gain health by providing abundant nutrients with relatively few calories. You'll find them well represented in the recipes in this book.

The other foods emphasized in the recipes come primarily from the Sonoma Diet tiered food lists that guide Sonoma Dieters in creating healthy meals to achieve weight loss. That means you can use these recipes to shed pounds (or to maintain the ideal weight you've achieved) while continuing with The Sonoma Diet.

Each recipe is designed so you can fill your Sonoma Diet plate or bowl with the proper amount of food in the healthiest proportions. Remember that the plate and bowl concept allows you to lose weight and gain health simply by eating the right foods in the right combination and the right amounts—without counting calories.

No More Diet Foods

What you won't find in this book are "low-carb" or "fat-free" restrictions that have been why so many weight loss plans fail long term. The Sonoma Diet emphasizes a healthy balance of all food types—including bread—from Day One. And that's why the recipes include beneficial carbohydrates such as whole grain breads and pastas and a variety of fruits and vegetables. You'll also enjoy taste-enhancing, heart-healthy fats such as olive oil, avocado, and nuts.

You'll find that the recipes and suggested side dishes in this book are strict about one thing—avoiding the kinds of carbs and fats that harm your health and sabotage your weight loss goals. Sugary foods and processed flour products such as white bread, crackers, regular pasta, and most (but not all) commercial cereals are no-no's on this diet. They won't even be mentioned in the pages that follow.

The same holds for the partially-hydrogenated trans fats and saturated fats. Unlike the unsaturated fats in olive oil and nuts, saturated fats, found mostly in animal and full-fat dairy and partially hydrogenated trans fats, increase your risk for heart disease and other diseases. They also bring with them high calorie counts that offer your body little in exchange except narrower arteries and a broader waistline. The recipes in this book limit saturated fats to the small acceptable levels found in otherwise healthy and nutritious foods, such as lean meat, and eliminate partially hydrogenated trans fats.

Just a Little for Flavor

Sharp-eyed Sonoma Diet veterans will notice that some of our recipes include ingredients not on the original Sonoma Diet food lists. For example, olives (a Sonoma County specialty) are often called for, but you won't find them on The Sonoma Diet vegetables list. The same is true for certain meats, such as prosciutto, and strong-flavored, aged cheeses, which are in some of these recipes but contain too much saturated fat to make The Sonoma Diet proteins list.

There's a reason for this seeming discrepancy. These foods serve as seasoning agents, not to fill a meal's quota of vegetables or protein. Small amounts of these foods go a long way to provide wonderful flavors. So think of these variations not as list crashers but as flavor enhancers. Use them like spices. As long as you apply them sparingly, they'll add variety to your meals.

Speaking of variety, here's one final word about the ingredients in The Sonoma Diet recipes. The emphasis is on a wide array of taste possibilities that make you look forward to each meal. But rest assured, there's nothing exotic about the recipes we're suggesting. Virtually all the ingredients you'll be using are found at your local supermarket. Every meal you'll be preparing will fit comfortably on just about any family's table. They're "different" only in that they're better tasting, healthier, and let you get rid of your extra pounds.

At the same time, you don't have to graduate from chef school to prepare these meals. The Sonoma Diet was created for people living in the real world, and so are the recipes in this book. Their goodness comes from wholesome, flavorful ingredients, not fancy cooking techniques.

Just as important, they don't require much time. Some are quicker than others, of course; that way you have the option of spending a little longer on a special dish. Or if you want a quick meal, look for the Sonoma Express icons. These recipes can be made in 30 minutes or less—including cooking time.

A NOTE ABOUT WAVE 3

If you've made it to Wave 3, congratulations! You've reached your weight loss goals and are ready to continue your healthy lifestyle. But if you're not sure exactly what to eat on Wave 3, here's a tip. Stick to the plate concept but allow yourself another serving of dairy, grain, and

fruit. This is the Wave where a little "heaping" on the plate (and an occasiaonal dessert) is okay. If you maintain your weight, you're on the right track. If you're gaining weight, cut back on your portions and refer back to the Tiers and the plate and bowl guidelines in The Sonoma Diet. And if you're still losing weight, up your portions or add some snacks. It may take a couple weeks to figure out what works best for your body. It may help to keep a journal of what changes you made from Wave 2 to help you as you continue Wave 3.

HOW TO USE THE BOOK

Just as the recipes are designed to be simple and self-explanatory, The Sonoma Diet Cookbook is organized for easy use. As you pick and choose among the meal ideas, keep the following features in mind:

• Each recipe includes a clear indication of which Sonoma Diet Wave (or Waves) it is appropriate for. That makes it easy for you to choose only those recipes that correspond to the Wave you're on. Once you're on Wave 3, of course, all recipes are allowed.

• Main dishes have "serve with" ideas to help you round out your Sonoma Diet plate. For instance, a main-dish beef recipe may offer a serving suggestion of a tossed salad if you're on Wave 1 and a salad, long grain brown rice, and fruit if you're on Wave 2 or 3. Note that these are only suggestions. Feel free to add your own sides, as long as they fit the plate concept and Sonoma food lists.

• The quickest-to-prepare meals are marked with an icon indicating a Sonoma Express recipe. That means they use a short list of ingredients and have a quick prep time. These are great for busy weeknights.

• As many Sonoma Dieters appreciate, a glass of wine with one daily meal on Waves 2 and 3 is allowed and encouraged. That's why there's a wine recommendation with each entrée. Not only does wine enhance the dining experience, it provides special antioxidants proven beneficial to overall health and longevity.

• Full nutrition information, including diabetic exchanges, is given for each recipe. This is not meant to say that The Sonoma Diet is appropriate for all diabetics. The exchanges are given to show how the recipes could fit in a diabetic diet that uses the American Diabetes Association's exchange system guidelines. Ask your physician or registered dietitian how the diet principles and recipes could work into your specific diabetic diet.

• Because holidays are challenging for many dieters, there's a special holiday section at the back of the book. Here you'll find festive meal ideas that don't stray from The Sonoma Diet tenets.

• Desserts and snacks are not prohibited on The Sonoma Diet, but only certain foods are allowed. A special chapter on desserts and snacks shows you how to find postmeal pleasure and between-meal satisfaction without slowing down your weight loss.

• None of the recipes are written in stone. There's plenty of room for tweaks and personal touches. In the following section, you'll find flavoring options and cooking techniques for adding personal variety to your meals. Remember that cooking for your own pleasure is part of the experience of The Sonoma Diet.

STAY IN SEASON

The Sonoma Diet encourages you to cook with produce that's currently growing in the fields. Those fruits and vegetables are at their peak flavor because they don't spend time in storage and they don't need to be artificially ripened after having been prematurely harvested.

Aim for these seasonal choices:

In spring choose artichokes, asparagus, beets, Blue Lake green beans, chard, arugula, mustard greens, morel mushrooms, peas, snap peas, snow peas, rhubarb, radishes, and zucchini.

In summer go for stone fruits, melons, berries, tomatoes, basil, green beans, shell beans, chard, corn, eggplant, peppers, porcini mushrooms, and summer squashes.

In fall your best choices are green beans, lima beans, apples, broccoli, broccoli rabe, Brussels sprouts, cabbages, cauliflower, celery root, chanterelle mushrooms, cranberries, fennel, figs, pears, persimmons, pomegranates, pumpkins, winter squashes, radicchio, and tangerines.

In winter in-season produce includes broccoli, Brussels sprouts, cabbages, celery root, winter squashes, citrus, escarole, endive, collard greens, mustard greens, parsnips, radicchio, and rutabaga.

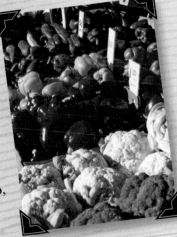

Adding Taste, Subtracting Pounds

Each recipe in **The Sonoma Diet Cookbook** is meant to give you more flavor and taste in your meals. Flavor and taste are actually two separate entities. Flavor is the aroma, texture, temperature, and often the beauty in foods. Taste is centered on the four sensations of bitter, sweet, salty, and sour. There is also a fifth taste, umami, which is described as the savory taste and satisfying aspect of certain foods. When combined with other tastes, umami creates a synergy that enhances the other flavors in foods. Umami is a taste based on natural compounds found in various foods such as mushrooms, almonds, red peppers, tomatoes, meats, aged cheese, soy sauce, olives, and broccoli. As you try the recipes in this book, be aware of the many different tastes and flavors in each bite.

20 FLAVOR BOOSTERS

You don't need expensive ingredients or fancy cooking techniques to get great-tasting foods. Try these ideas to capture the flavor and health in wholesome foods.

1. Spice rubs, pastes, and marinades
Spice rubs are a quick, dry alternative to marinades. Used to coat meat with flavor, rubs are usually a blend of herbs, spices, and other seasonings, sometimes made into a paste by adding oil.

2. Powders
You'll find them made from mushrooms, vegetables, garlic, olives—even fruit.

3. Pan drippings
This is the concentrated bits of flavor that remain in the saucepan after you sauté or roast an item.

4. Glazes
Glazes are glossy, rich mixtures used to coat meats or vegetables. Sometimes it may be a jelled broth or reduced liquid, such as fruit or vegetable juice, which adds the final touch to a simple dish.

5. Chile peppers
Dry or fresh. There are lots of varieties to choose from.

6. Vegetables
Roasted or grilled, they can serve as flavor enhancers.

7. Salsas
An endless source of taste turners, bottled or fresh.

8. Chutneys
Made from vegetables, fruits, or beans, they are a great accompaniment to meat and poultry.

9. Full-flavored oils
Try sesame, walnut, almond, and extra-virgin olive oil. Drizzle on a finished dish to add flavor and richness.

10. Infused oils and vinegars
The flavor opportunities increase when oils or vinegars are permeated with herbs and/or fruits. Use in marinades, vinaigrettes, and dressings.

11. Sun-dried foods
Tomatoes, of course, but also cherries, cranberries, raisins, and mushrooms. Use a little to add texture and flavor to pastas, salads, stuffings, and sauces.

12. Full-flavored and dried, aged cheeses
Try pecorino, Parmesan, goat cheese, Gorgonzola, and feta cheese. Just a little goes a long way on a finished dish.

13. Pickled, cured, and brined ingredients
Try capers, pepperoncinis, anchovies, and olives. You only need a small amount of these salty and intensely flavored taste inhansers in a recipe. Too much can overpower a dish.

14. Aromatics
Ginger, garlic, green onions, and shallots; These ingredients create a flavor base for sauteed items, marinades, vinaigrettes, and sauces.

15. Bean water
The liquid in which beans are cooked is flavor rich and full of body. Use this in place of water or stock in dishes that contain beans. It can add body to an otherwise thin sauce.

16. Seeds and nuts
Roast them first for extra flavor.

17. Cooked vegetables or fruit purees
A puree of roasted red bell peppers can add color and flavor to grilled fish or chicken. A fruit puree can be the sauce for many desserts.

18. Wood chips
For tastier grilled foods, add soaked wood chips made from oak, mesquite, grape vines, cherry wood, pecan wood, or maple wood. Add sprigs of rosemary, sage, thyme, or lavender to the fire for aroma and flavor.

19. Dry herbs with oil
To bring out the most flavor in dry herbs, gently heat them first in a little oil. Infused into the oil, the aromatic ingredients come to life.

20. Toasted spices
Putting them in a dry pan over low heat brings out the resinous oils in spices and jump-starts their flavor-enhancing abilities.

Be Salt Savvy

Salt's role in cooking is to turn up the flavor, not to turn food taste "salty." Used correctly, it will make your meats taste meatier and bring out the natural taste of your ingredients. Here are some suggestions for salting.

Choose the right salt. There are many different types of salt available, but not all are created equal. For everyday cooking, try kosher salt, instead of traditional table salt. Kosher salt is a pure mined salt with a flake shape, not granular or cubed. It has a clean taste and dissolves clearly in food.

Sea salts are great for finishing a dish. They come in a variety of flavors and textures. For a quick side dish, sprinkle coarse sea salt on vine-ripe tomatoes, then drizzle with extra-virgin olive oil and a little basil.

Salt as you cook. If you wait until the end of cooking, you'll get a superficial salt flavor, with the rest of the ingredients tasting bland.

Salt meats prior to cooking them. This will not dry out the meat. Instead, the meat's juices will mix with the salt and will be drawn back into the meat. That's what gives meat its full flavor. Lightly salt the meat prior to placing in a marinade or before using a rub or paste.

Season liquids when cooking pilafs. In fact, the broth should almost seem a little too salty at first when you cook a grain pilaf-style. The grain or rice itself will dilute the salt flavor by the time the liquid is absorbed. Plus, when cooking pilaf in pre-salted (and -seasoned) liquid, you shouldn't have to stir the delicate cooked grains before serving.

Salt and cooking beans. This is an exception to cooking with salt. Early salting toughens the skin on beans, so they take longer to cook. Always salt beans when they're almost cooked through to flavor the entire bean.

Flavor for Free

The goal of healthy cooking is to capture "free" flavor—the aromatic natural goodness in foods that brings taste without extra calories or harmful additives. Use the following techniques to bring out the free flavor in food:

Sweating. This simply refers to cooking vegetables very slowly to concentrate their flavor. Cook them over low heat in a covered pan until they're translucent and meltingly tender. Do this by adding very little oil, a tablespoon of water, whichever herbs or spices you choose, and a pinch of salt to your vegetables.

Poaching: Poaching is cooking in a flavored liquid at a much lower temperature than simmering, with the liquid barely moving. This slow, gentle poach keeps whatever you're cooking tender. Anything hotter will yield a tough and rubbery piece of meat, chicken, or seafood. Make sure that the poaching liquid is fully flavored. Use vegetable stock or a juice and add aromatic herbs and spices.

Caramelization. This is a fancy word for browning the exterior of whatever you're cooking. There are lots of techniques for it, including grilling, sauteing, braising, and roasting.

Sauteing. It's the surest and easiest technique for getting a nice brown, caramelized surface. To get the brown surface you want from sauteing, you need a hot pan so that the food starts browning immediately; otherwise, it will just sit there oozing liquid and turn tough. So heat your saute pan for 30 seconds to a minute before adding oil. You'll know the pan is hot enough if a drop of water skitters and then evaporates immediately. Once the meat is caramelized, turn down the heat. When sauteing onions, make sure they get translucent and slightly golden.

Searing. You will want to sear meat prior to cooking with a flavored liquid (braising). Essentially, searing means sauteing briefly on all sides in a very hot pan before adding liquid and letting the food simmer until tender. Searing ensures a rich, full-bodied flavor with a meaty sauce, as well as a tender texture.

Roasting. Both meat and vegetables can be roasted for a special flavor. Make sure you pre-heat the oven before you put anything into it. When roasting vegetables, season them, then spread them out in a single layer, turning them periodically during roasting. That way they will roast and not steam.

FAVORITES FOR YOUR SONOMA DIET KITCHEN

Live The Sonoma Diet way by stocking your kitchen with these healthy and flavorful foods.

1. Fresh Herbs. They offer the gift of bright, full flavors with minimal calories. There are actually two classes of herbs—fine and resinous.

Fine herbs are tenderer due to a higher water content and are usually bright, fresh, and grassy. Examples are basil, cilantro, chervil, dill, parsley, and tarragon. Their stems are tender, so it's okay if you chop them up with the leaves. They're best with minimal cooking, so add them to dishes later in the cooking process. And, much like lettuce, their whole leaves are good in salads and sandwiches.

Resinous herbs are chewier with a higher oil content. They have tough stems, so you need to get rid of them. The leaves can be chewy, so finely chop them. Familiar resinous herbs are rosemary, thyme, marjoram, oregano, and bay leaves. They benefit from a longer cooking time, so add resinous herbs to the onions and garlic at the beginning of the cooking process.

If necessary, you can substitute dried herbs for fresh herbs using about one-third the amount. Treat dry herbs like resinous herbs, adding them early in the cooking process.

2. Spices. Keep a variety of your favorite spices—whole and ground—on hand. Must-haves are caraway seeds, coriander seeds, cumin, black peppercorns, fennel seeds, cinnamon, star anise, and Spanish paprika. Don't use spices more than a year old. Buy them from a quality source that goes through its stock quickly.

3. Aromatic Vegetables. Onions and garlic come to mind first in this category. They're a wonderful base for just about any Mediterranean dish. But carrots and celery also qualify. Carrots add sweetness, and celery adds its own unique flavor. Sweat carrots and celery in oil for a light color and delicate flavor in your dish. Or caramelize them for a dark brown color and deep, rich flavor.

4. Beans. They offer fiber, protein, and a satisfying sense of fullness. Garbanzos, white beans, black beans, pinto beans, and cannellini beans make a good starting lineup. Keep cans of cooked beans in your pantry for those days when you don't have time to cook them yourself.

5. Whole Grains and Lentils. Use quinoa, coarse bulgur and green or black lentils. They're quick and easy to prepare. Changing the spices and herbs you cook them with adds variety. Try them in combination with beans or toss a handful in salads.

6. Extra-Virgin Olive Oil. Keep two types of extra-virgin olive oil in your pantry. One will be for cooking, the other for "finishing."

The oil you'll use for sauteing, roasting, grilling, marinades, and vinaigrettes should have a good, clean flavor but be able to take high heat. It will generally be less expensive.

Use the other oil to enhance finished dishes or to add to salads. Drizzle a little over a bowl of lentil soup just before serving or over spinach in an already lightly dressed salad. This bottle of extra-virgin olive oil should be strong on flavor.

7. Acids. Always keep a few fresh lemons and a variety of vinegars on hand. Recommended vinegars include balsamic, red wine, white wine, and sherry. Quality is essential here because cheap generic vinegars get their color from dyes and have a sharp or harsh edge. Choose a name brand in the midprice range.

8. Nuts. Keep a variety handy. Almonds, walnuts, pine nuts, and peanuts are best. Store raw nuts in the refrigerator to help keep their oils from turning rancid. Toasting adds flavor, but don't toast them in a saute pan on the stove. They'll often come out burnt on the outside and raw on the inside. Instead, place nuts (of similar size) in a single layer on a baking sheet and put them in a 350°F oven for five to 10 minutes.

9. Condiments. Full-flavored mustard (like whole grain or Dijon), horseradish, canned chipotle chiles in adobo, Chinese black bean sauce, and hot sauces are ingredients with minimal calories and lots of flavor. Stir in a spoonful of Chinese black bean sauce when simmering grains or beans for a stir-fry. Serve horseradish with beef or add to a sauce.

10. Cheese. You want strongly-flavored cheeses, where a little goes a long way. Keep a small wedge of a good Grana Padana or Parmigiano-Reggiano cheese in your refrigerator, along with a small piece of feta and Asiago. These are always welcome additions to a salad or whole-grain pasta. Go for quality. There's a huge difference between fresh Parmesan cheese and the packaged store brand. You'll get more flavor with less, saving money and calories.

11. Sun-dried, Cured, and Pickled Ingredients. Capers, olives, pepperoncinis, roasted peppers, roasted garlic, sun-dried tomatoes, dried mushrooms, and anchovies just to name a few. These are high-flavor-impact ingredients, many of which are high in umami. The addition of a small amount of these ingredients will add dimension and flavor to any recipe. Add a few capers and chopped olives to a simple pasta dish or salad. Add dried mushrooms to a sauce to give it depth and umami.

SLOW DOWN AND SAVOR EACH BITE

One last tip before you explore the culinary treats ahead: Once you've prepared any of these Sonoma Diet meals, take the time to savor it. Slow, leisurely meals that stimulate all the senses are a hallmark of The Sonoma Diet style. They're also the best way to experience these healthy, wholesome recipes. On The Sonoma Diet, mealtime pleasure isn't just a bonus. It's a weight loss strategy that becomes part of a lifestyle.

Enjoy your meals!

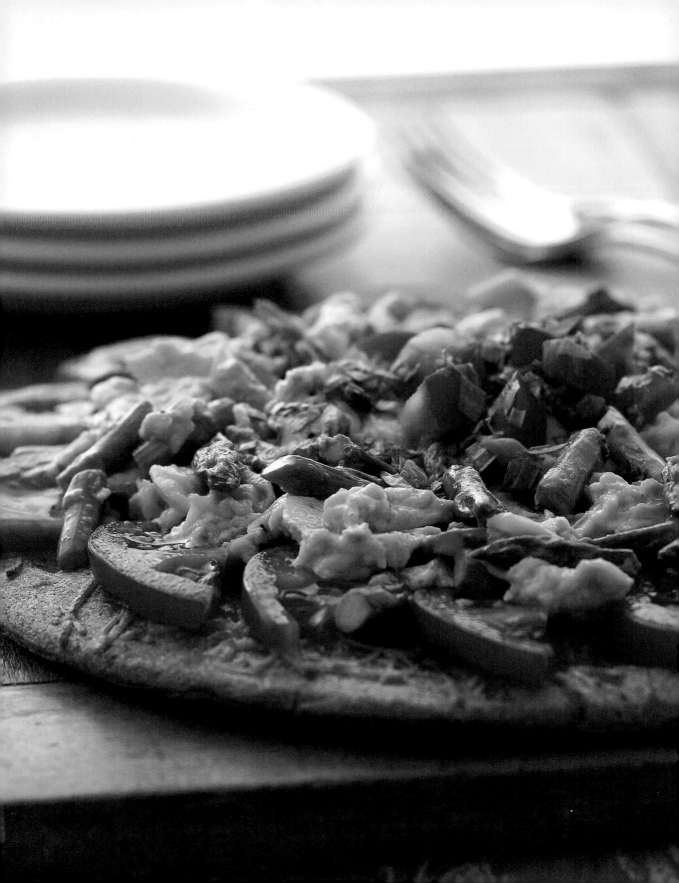

Breakfast Sonoma-Style

Morning meals don't have to be limited to cereal or scrambled eggs. Get creative with these delicious a.m. treats. Don't let those Mediterranean names scare you. These quiches, stratas, frittatas, and casseroles are a snap to cook. You can even prepare some in advance, then heat them up in the morning as the coffee brews.

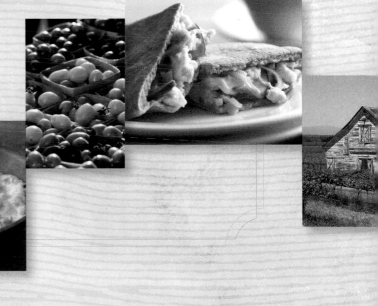

CRUSTLESS FETA AND CHEDDAR QUICHE

*The mingling of cheeses in this savory quiche gives it a full,
rich flavor you'll want to let linger on your taste buds.*

Prep: 25 minutes **Bake:** 40 minutes **Oven:** 350°F **Makes:** 8 servings

Nonstick olive oil cooking spray

4 beaten eggs

⅓ cup whole wheat pastry flour

4 cloves garlic, minced (2 teaspoons minced)

1 tablespoon chopped fresh dillweed, thyme, or mint

¼ teaspoon freshly ground black pepper

⅛ teaspoon kosher salt

1½ cups low-fat cottage cheese (12 ounces)

1 10-ounce package frozen chopped broccoli, cooked and drained

1 cup crumbled feta cheese (4 ounces)

1 cup shredded reduced-fat cheddar cheese (4 ounces)

1. Preheat oven to 350°F. Lightly coat a 9-inch pie plate with cooking spray.

2. In a medium bowl combine eggs, pastry flour, garlic, dillweed, pepper, and kosher salt. Stir in cottage cheese, broccoli, feta, and cheddar. Spoon into the pie prepared plate.

3. Bake for 40 to 45 minutes or until a knife inserted near center comes out clean. Cool on a wire rack for 5 to 10 minutes before serving.

Nutrition facts per serving: 188 cal., 10 g total fat (6 g sat. fat), 134 mg chol., 575 mg sodium, 9 g carbo., 2 g fiber, 16 g pro.
Exchanges: ½ Vegetable, ½ Starch, 2 Lean Meat, ½ Fat

For Waves 1, 2, and 3, serve with whole grain toast.

Olive Oil   *Whole Grains*

Broccoli

VEGETABLE QUICHES

This version of the classic French dish eliminates the high-fat pastry
while maintaining beneficial nutrients and delicious flavor.

Prep: 25 minutes **Bake:** 25 minutes **Stand:** 5 minutes **Oven:** 375°F **Makes:** 6 servings

Nonstick olive oil cooking spray

3 7- or 8-inch whole wheat flour tortillas

2 ounces reduced-fat Swiss, cheddar, or mozzarella cheese, shredded (½ cup)

1 cup broccoli florets

½ of a small red bell pepper, cut into thin bite-size strips

4 eggs

¾ cup evaporated fat-free milk

¼ teaspoon dried thyme, crushed

⅛ teaspoon kosher salt

⅛ teaspoon freshly ground black pepper

Thin strips red bell pepper (optional)

Olive Oil

Bell Peppers

Broccoli

Whole Grains

1. Preheat oven to 375°F. Coat six 6- to 7-inch individual round baking dishes or pans° with nonstick cooking spray. Carefully press tortillas into dishes or pans. Sprinkle with cheese.

2. In a small covered saucepan cook the broccoli and bell pepper strips in a small amount of boiling water about 3 minutes or until crisp-tender. Drain well. Sprinkle cooked vegetables over cheese in baking dishes.

3. In a medium bowl whisk together eggs, evaporated fat-free milk, thyme, kosher salt, and black pepper until well mixed. Pour egg mixture over vegetables in baking dishes. Place on baking sheet.

4. Bake for 25 to 30 minutes or until puffed and a knife inserted near center of each comes out clean. Let stand for 5 minutes before serving. If desired, garnish with additional strips of bell pepper.

Nutrition facts per serving: 185 cal., 8 g total fat (3 g sat. fat), 151 mg chol., 314 mg sodium, 13 g carbo., 6 g fiber, 15 g pro.
Exchanges: ½ Vegetable, ½ Starch, 2 Medium-Fat Meat

*Note: Or coat six 6-ounce custard cups with nonstick cooking spray. Cut each tortilla into 6 wedges. To form crust, press 3 tortilla wedges into each custard cup with points toward center. Tortillas do not have to cover cups completely. Continue as directed.

For Waves 1, 2, and 3, serve as is.

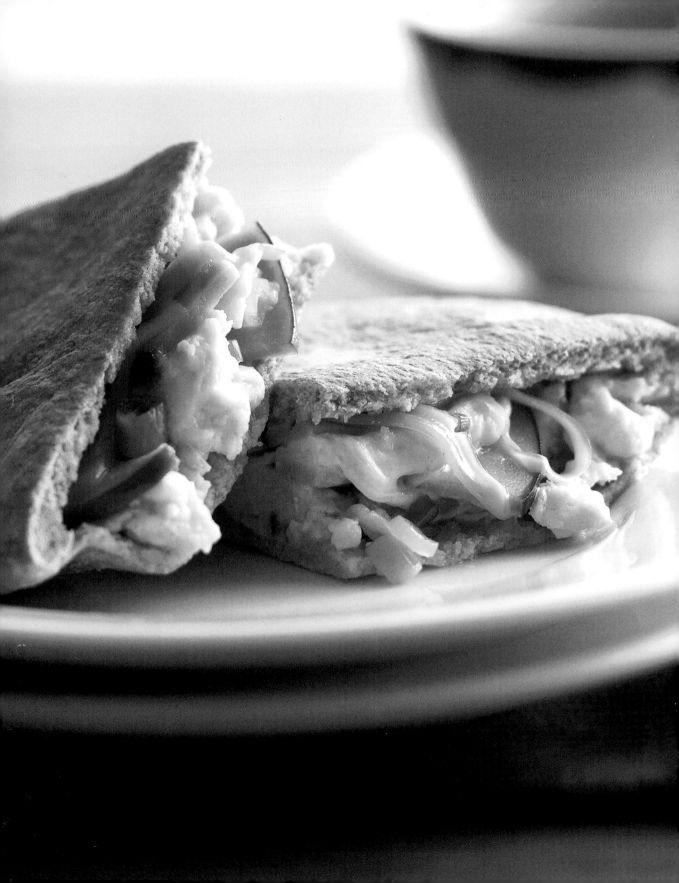

CANADIAN BACON AND EGG POCKETS

Enjoy this simple sandwich-style breakfast and you'll meet both your grain and protein recommendations to start your morning off right. Canadian-style bacon is a leaner alternative to bacon, yet gives the dish intensified flavor.

Start to Finish: 15 minutes **Makes:** 4 servings

4 egg whites

2 eggs

3 tablespoons water

⅛ teaspoon kosher salt

3 ounces Canadian-style bacon, chopped

2 tablespoons sliced green onion (optional)

Nonstick olive oil cooking spray

2 large whole wheat pita bread rounds, halved crosswise

2 ounces reduced-fat cheddar cheese, shredded (½ cup) (optional)

Olive Oil

Whole Grains

1. In a medium bowl combine egg whites, eggs, water, and salt. Beat with a wire whisk or rotary beater until well mixed. Stir in Canadian bacon and, if desired, green onion.

2. Lightly coat an unheated large nonstick skillet with nonstick cooking spray. Preheat over medium heat. Add egg mixture to skillet. Cook, without stirring, until mixture begins to set on the bottom and around edge.

3. Using a spatula or a large spoon, lift and fold the partially cooked eggs so the uncooked portion flows underneath. Continue cooking for about 2 minutes or until egg mixture is cooked through but is still glossy and moist. Remove from heat immediately.

4. Open pita halves to form a pocket. Fill pita halves with egg mixture. If desired, sprinkle with cheese.

Nutrition facts per serving: 162 cal., 4 g total fat (1 g sat. fat), 118 mg chol., 616 mg sodium, 18 g carbo., 2 g fiber, 13 g pro.
Exchanges: 1 Starch, 1½ Very Lean Meat, ½ Fat

For Waves 1, 2, and 3, serve as is.

BREAKFAST TORTILLA WRAP

Make this quick-to-the-table dish as spicy or mild as you like by adding or omitting the crushed red pepper and adobo sauce. Whichever way you choose, you'll be getting healthful benefits from the green peppers and tomatoes—two of the Sonoma Top 10 Power Foods.

Start to Finish: 15 minutes **Makes:** 1 serving

1   slice Canadian-style bacon, chopped

1   teaspoon extra-virgin olive oil

2   tablespoons chopped green bell pepper

⅛   teaspoon kosher salt

⅛   teaspoon ground cumin

⅛   teaspoon crushed red pepper (optional)

2   slightly beaten egg whites

2   tablespoons chopped tomato

    Few dashes bottled adobo or other hot pepper sauce (optional)

1   8-inch whole wheat flour tortilla, warmed

1. In a medium nonstick skillet cook Candian-style bacon just until starting to brown. Add olive oil; heat. Add bell pepper, kosher salt, cumin, and, if desired, crushed red pepper. Cook for 3 minutes. Add egg whites; cook for 2 minutes. Stir in tomato and, if desired, adobo sauce. Spoon onto tortilla and roll up.

Nutrition facts per serving: 239 cal., 9 g total fat (2 g sat. fat), 15 mg chol., 1,054 mg sodium, 17 g carbo., 11 g fiber, 21 g pro.
Exchanges: 1 Starch, 2½ Very Lean Meat, 1½ Fat

For Waves 1, 2, and 3, serve as is.

Olive Oil

Bell Peppers

Tomatoes

Whole Grains

SOUTHWEST BREAKFAST STRATA

The word "strata" refers to many layers. This multilayered, brightly colored dish is loaded with flavor boosters to give your taste buds a wake-up call.

Prep: 15 minutes **Chill:** 4 to 24 hours **Bake:** 25 minutes **Oven:** 350°F **Makes:** 6 servings

Nonstick olive oil cooking spray

6 slices whole wheat bread, dried

6 eggs

2 tablespoons canned diced green chile peppers

⅛ teaspoon freshly ground black pepper

2 slices Canadian-style bacon, cut into thin strips, or ½ cup chopped cooked ham

2 roma tomatoes, thinly sliced

2 ounces reduced-fat Monterey Jack cheese, shredded (½ cup)

1 tablespoon chopped fresh cilantro

1. Lightly coat a 2-quart rectangular baking dish with nonstick cooking spray. Cover the bottom of the prepared baking dish with bread slices, cutting to fit.

2. In a medium bowl whisk together eggs, chile peppers, and black pepper until well mixed. Pour egg mixture evenly over bread. Sprinkle with Canadian-style bacon or ham. Top with sliced tomato and cheese. Cover and refrigerate 4 to 24 hours.

3. Preheat oven to 350°F. Bake, uncovered, about 25 minutes or until a knife inserted near center comes out clean. Sprinkle with cilantro.

Nutrition facts per serving: 181 cal., 9 g total fat (3 g sat. fat), 223 mg chol., 428 mg sodium, 13 g carbo., 2 g fiber, 13 g pro.
Exchanges: 1 Starch, 1½ Medium-Fat Meat

For Waves 1, 2, and 3, serve as is.

Olive Oil　　*Whole Grains*

Tomatoes

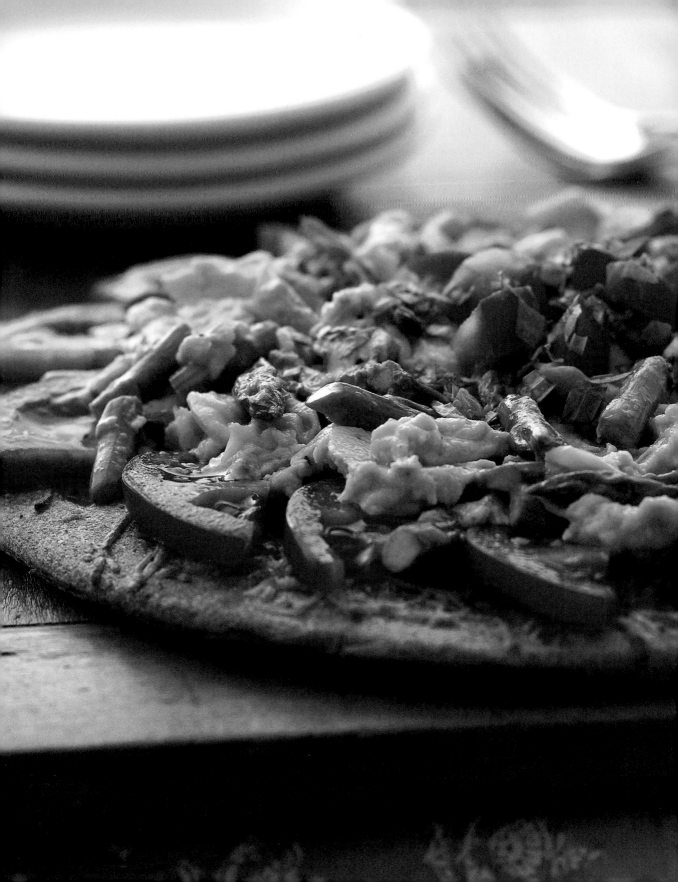

TOMATO AND ASPARAGUS PIZZA

With this unique dish, flash back to the days when pizza for breakfast was commonplace. The inclusion of tomatoes, asparagus, garlic, and herbs ensures you get plenty of vitamins and beneficial phytochemicals.

Start to Finish: 20 minutes **Oven:** 450°F **Makes:** 6 servings

1   12-inch whole wheat Italian bread shell (such as Boboli brand)

6   eggs

⅓   cup low-fat milk

2   teaspoons chopped fresh tarragon or oregano

⅛   teaspoon kosher salt

⅛   teaspoon freshly ground black pepper

1   cup fresh asparagus bias-cut into 1-inch pieces

1   clove garlic, minced (½ teaspoon minced)

1   tablespoon extra-virgin olive oil

1   large tomato, halved and sliced

Chopped fresh tomato (optional)

Chopped fresh tarragon (optional)

1. Preheat oven to 450°F. Place bread shell on a 12-inch pizza pan. Bake for 8 to 10 minutes or until heated through.

2. Meanwhile, in a medium bowl beat together eggs, milk, 2 teaspoons tarragon, kosher salt, and pepper. In a large nonstick skillet cook asparagus and garlic in hot oil over medium heat for 3 minutes; pour egg mixture over asparagus mixture in skillet. Cook over medium heat, without stirring, until mixture begins to set on the bottom and around edge.

3. Using a spatula, lift and fold the partially cooked egg mixture so the uncooked portion flows underneath. Continue cooking for 2 to 3 minutes or until egg mixture is cooked through but is still glossy and moist. Remove from heat immediately.

4. Arrange tomato slices evenly around the edge of the baked bread shell. Spoon scrambled egg mixture in the center. If desired, garnish with additional chopped tomato and tarragon. Cut into wedges; serve immediately.

Nutrition facts per serving: 234 cal., 10 g total fat (2 g sat. fat), 212 mg chol., 376 mg sodium, 26 g carbo., 4 g fiber, 13 g pro.
Exchanges: ½ Vegetable, 1½ Starch, 1 Medium-Fat Meat, ½ Fat

For Waves 1, 2, and 3, serve as is.

Olive Oil

Whole Grains

Tomatoes

BAKED BRIE STRATA

*Brie, acclaimed as one of the world's greatest cheeses, gives this delectable dish a robust flavor.
If you prefer, assemble this strata the night before so it's ready for baking the next morning.*

Prep: 25 minutes **Chill:** 4 to 24 hours **Bake:** 55 minutes **Stand:** 10 minutes **Oven:** 325°F **Makes:** 6 servings

2   small zucchini, cut crosswise into ¼-inch-thick slices (about 2 cups)

⅛   teaspoon kosher salt

⅛   teaspoon freshly ground black pepper

    Nonstick olive oil cooking spray

6   slices whole wheat bread, dried and torn into bite-size pieces

1   4.4-ounce package Brie cheese, cut into ½-inch cubes

1   cup halved grape or cherry tomatoes

4   eggs

⅔   cup evaporated fat-free milk

⅓   cup sliced green onions

3   tablespoons chopped fresh dill

½   teaspoon kosher salt

⅛   teaspoon freshly ground black pepper

Olive Oil

Whole Grains

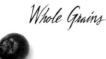

Tomatoes

1. In a covered medium saucepan cook zucchini in a small amount of boiling lightly salted water for 2 to 3 minutes or just until tender. Drain zucchini; transfer to a medium bowl. Season with ⅛ teaspoon kosher salt and pepper. Set aside.

2. Meanwhile, coat a 2-quart rectangular baking dish with nonstick cooking spray. Arrange 4 cups of the bread pieces in the prepared baking dish. If desired, remove and discard rind from cheese. Sprinkle cheese evenly over bread in baking dish. Arrange zucchini and tomatoes on top. Sprinkle with remaining 2 cups bread pieces.

3. In a medium bowl whisk together eggs, evaporated fat-free milk, green onions, dill, kosher salt, and pepper. Pour evenly over mixture in baking dish. Lightly press down layers with back of spoon. Cover with plastic wrap; chill for 4 to 24 hours.

4. Preheat oven to 325°F. Remove plastic wrap from strata; cover with foil. Bake for 30 minutes. Uncover; bake for 25 to 30 minutes more or until a knife inserted near the center comes out clean. Let stand for 10 minutes before serving.

Nutrition facts per serving: 216 cal., 10 g total fat
(5 g sat. fat), 163 mg chol., 549 mg sodium, 18 g carbo.,
3 g fiber, 14 g pro.
Exchanges: ½ Vegetable, 1 Starch, 1½ Medium-Fat
Meat, 1 Fat

For Waves 1, 2, and 3, serve as is.

BREAKFAST CASSEROLE

Enjoy all your favorite breakfast flavors—sausage, eggs, and cheese—in this one-dish meal.

Prep: 25 minutes **Chill:** 2 to 24 hours **Bake:** 32 minutes **Stand:** 5 minutes **Oven:** 350°F **Makes:** 8 servings

6 slices whole wheat bread
   Nonstick olive oil cooking spray

4 ounces bulk turkey sausage

1 medium red or green bell pepper, chopped

½ cup chopped fresh mushrooms

2 ounces reduced-fat sharp cheddar
   cheese, shredded (½ cup)

1 10¾-ounce can reduced-fat and
   reduced-sodium condensed cream of
   mushroom soup

4 beaten eggs

1 cup evaporated fat-free milk

¾ teaspoon dry mustard

¼ teaspoon freshly ground black pepper

1. Preheat oven to 350°F. Cut bread into cubes; place in a large shallow pan. Bake for 8 to 10 minutes or until toasted, stirring once. Coat a 2-quart rectangular baking dish with nonstick cooking spray. Place half of the toasted bread cubes in the dish. Set aside.

2. Meanwhile, in a large skillet cook sausage, bell pepper, and mushrooms over medium-high heat until sausage is brown. Drain off fat. Pat mixture with paper towels to remove excess fat. Spoon mixture over bread cubes in dish. Sprinkle with half of the cheese. Top with remaining bread.

3. In a medium bowl combine soup, eggs, evaporated fat-free milk, dry mustard, and black pepper. Pour over bread, pressing down cubes with back of spoon to moisten. Cover and refrigerate for 2 to 24 hours.

4. Bake, uncovered, about 30 minutes or until a knife inserted near the center comes out clean. Sprinkle with remaining cheese. Bake for 2 to 3 minutes more. Remove from oven. Let stand for 5 to 10 minutes before serving.

Nutrition facts per serving: 179 cal., 6 g total fat (3 g sat. fat), 124 mg chol., 458 mg sodium, 17 g carbo., 2 g fiber, 12 g pro.
Exchanges: 1 Starch, 1 Lean Meat, ½ Fat

For Waves 1, 2, and 3, serve as is.

Olive Oil

Whole Grains

Bell Peppers

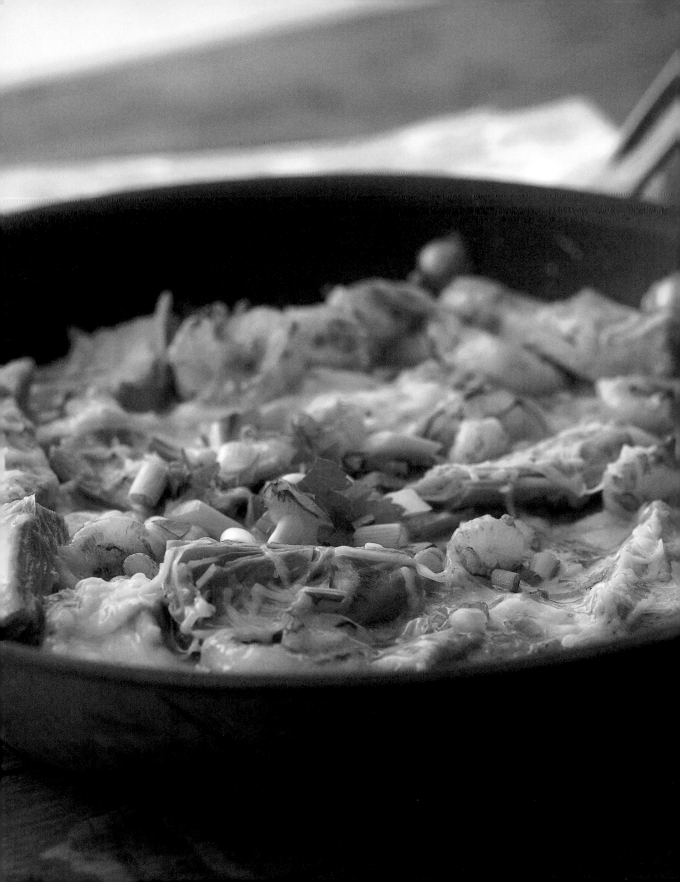

SHRIMP-ARTICHOKE FRITTATA

*Add some crustacean character to your basic frittata by including shrimp,
a great source of tryptophan and selenium.*

Start to Finish: 25 minutes **Makes:** 4 servings

4   ounces fresh or frozen shrimp in shells

Kosher salt

Freshly ground black pepper

½   of a 9-ounce package frozen artichoke hearts

8   eggs

¼   cup fat-free or low-fat milk

¼   cup thinly sliced green onions

⅛   teaspoon garlic powder

⅛   teaspoon freshly ground black pepper

Nonstick olive oil cooking spray

3   tablespoons finely shredded Parmesan cheese

Sliced green onions (optional)

Fresh flat-leaf parsley (optional)

Olive Oil

1. Thaw shrimp, if frozen. Peel and devein shrimp. Rinse shrimp; pat dry with paper towels. Halve shrimp lengthwise; season shrimp with kosher salt and pepper. Set aside. Meanwhile, cook artichoke hearts according to package directions; drain. Cut artichoke hearts into quarters; season lightly with kosher salt and pepper. Set aside.

2. In a large bowl whisk together eggs, milk, ¼ cup green onions, the garlic powder, and the ⅛ teaspoon pepper; set aside.

3. Lightly coat an unheated large nonstick skillet with nonstick cooking spray. Preheat over medium heat. Add shrimp to hot skillet; cook shrimp for 1 to 3 minutes or until shrimp are opaque. Reduce heat to medium-low.

4. Pour egg mixture into skillet; do not stir. As the egg mixture sets, run a spatula around the edge of the skillet, lifting egg mixture so uncooked portion flows underneath. Continue cooking and lifting edges until egg mixture is almost set (surface will be moist).

5. Remove skillet from heat; sprinkle artichoke pieces evenly over the top. Sprinkle with Parmesan cheese. Cover and let stand for 3 to 4 minutes or until top is set. Loosen edge of frittata. Transfer to a serving plate; cut into wedges to serve. If desired, garnish with additional sliced green onions and fresh parsley.

Nutrition facts per serving: 301 cal., 17 g total fat
(8 g sat. fat), 484 mg chol., 809 mg sodium, 6 g carbo.,
1 g fiber, 29 g pro.
Exchanges: ½ Vegetable, 1 Very Lean Meat, 3 Medium-
Fat Meat, ½ Fat

*For Waves 1, 2, and 3, serve with whole
grain toast.*

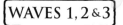 TOMATO AND BASIL FRITTATA

Loaded with nutrients and phytochemicals, this egg-based dish includes basil, a key herb in Mediterranean cooking, for enhanced flavor.

Prep: 15 minutes **Bake:** 7 minutes **Oven:** 350°F **Makes:** 2 servings

5   egg whites

1   egg

1   tablespoon chopped fresh basil or
    ½ teaspoon dried basil, crushed

⅛   teaspoon kosher salt

    Dash freshly ground black pepper

    Nonstick olive oil cooking spray

1   cup chopped fresh spinach

2   green onions, sliced

1   clove garlic, minced (½ teaspoon minced)

1   small tomato, chopped

1   ounce reduced-fat cheddar cheese,
    shredded (¼ cup)

1. Preheat oven to 350°F. In a medium bowl lightly beat together egg whites and whole egg. Stir in basil, kosher salt, and pepper; set aside.

2. Coat an unheated 8-inch oven-going skillet with nonstick cooking spray. Preheat the skillet over medium heat. Add spinach, green onions, and garlic. Cook for 1 to 2 minutes or until spinach begins to wilt. Remove skillet from heat; drain, if necessary.

3. Pour egg mixture over spinach mixture in the skillet. Bake for 6 to 8 minutes or until eggs are set. Sprinkle with chopped tomato and cheese. Bake for 1 to 2 minutes more or until the cheese melts. Cut the frittata into wedges to serve.

Nutrition facts per serving: 138 cal., 6 g total fat (3 g sat. fat), 116 mg chol., 425 mg sodium, 5 g carbo., 1 g fiber, 17 g pro.
Exchanges: 1 Vegetable, 2 Lean Meat

For Waves 1, 2, and 3, serve with whole grain toast.

Olive Oil

Spinach

Tomatoes

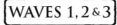
VEGETABLE FRITTATA

Broccoli, carrots, and basil create a vibrant mosaic for your breakfast plate.
The many colors of this dish reflect its high antioxidant content.

Start to Finish: 25 minutes **Makes:** 8 servings

1 cup water

1 cup broccoli florets

½ cup finely chopped carrot

¼ cup sliced green onions

Kosher salt

Freshly ground black pepper

Nonstick olive oil cooking spray

¾ cup shredded reduced-fat cheddar or Swiss cheese (3 ounces)

8 eggs

1 tablespoon chopped fresh basil or 1 teaspoon dried basil, crushed

1 tablespoon Dijon-style mustard

¼ teaspoon freshly ground black pepper

Tomato slices (optional)

Olive Oil

Broccoli

1. In a medium saucepan combine the water, broccoli, carrot, and green onions. Bring to boiling; reduce heat. Cover and simmer for 6 to 8 minutes or until vegetables are crisp-tender. Drain well. Transfer to a medium bowl and season lightly with kosher salt and pepper.

2. Coat an unheated large nonstick skillet with nonstick cooking spray. Spread the cooked vegetables in the bottom of the skillet. Sprinkle with half of the cheese. In a medium bowl whisk together eggs, basil, mustard, and the ¼ teaspoon pepper. Pour over vegetables and cheese in skillet. Cook over medium heat. As egg mixture sets, run a spatula around the edge of the skillet, lifting egg mixture so the uncooked portion flows underneath. Continue cooking and lifting the edge until egg mixture is almost set (surface will be moist). Remove from heat.

3. Cover and let stand for 3 to 4 minutes or until top is set. To serve, cut the frittata into wedges. Sprinkle with the remaining cheese. If desired, garnish with tomato slices.

Nutrition facts per serving: 114 cal., 7 g total fat (3 g sat. fat), 219 mg chol., 245 mg sodium, 3 g carbo., 1 g fiber, 10 g pro.
Exchanges: ½ Vegetable, 1½ Medium-Fat Meat

For Waves 1, 2, and 3, serve with whole grain toast.

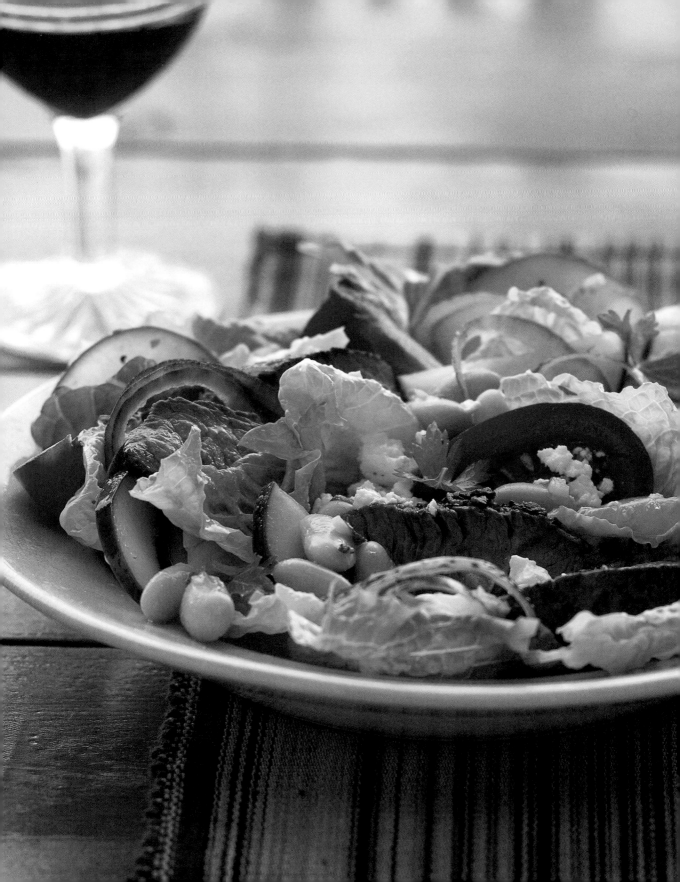

Soups, Salads & Sandwiches

When you want something that's quick to make for dinner or when you want a really great lunch, you'll want to try these recipes. You'll find soups filled with nutty grains, sandwiches filled with lean meats, and fresh herbs and salads brimming with crunchy produce. Flavorful spices and easy-to-find ingredients turn these simple meals into wonderfully satisfying experiences.

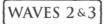
SPICY CHICKEN AND HOMINY STEW

This Southwestern-style soup uses green salsa to really heat things up.
If spicy isn't your style, stick to the low end of the range for the salsa.

Prep: 25 minutes **Cook:** 10 minutes **Makes:** 6 servings

1   tablespoon extra-virgin olive oil

1   pound skinless, boneless chicken breast halves, cut into 1-inch cubes

1½   cups chopped red onion

6   cloves garlic, minced (1 tablespoon minced)

2   15-ounce cans hominy, rinsed and drained

2   14-ounce cans reduced-sodium chicken broth

1   cup pitted ripe olives, quartered

½   to 1 cup purchased green salsa or green enchilada sauce*

¼   cup finely chopped red bell pepper

¼   cup chopped fresh cilantro

½   of an avocado, seeded, peeled, and chopped (optional)

2   tablespoons fat-free dairy sour cream (optional)

2   tablespoons grated cotija cheese or finely shredded mozzarella cheese (optional)

1. In a 4-quart Dutch oven heat olive oil over medium-high heat. Add chicken; cook and stir for 3 to 4 minutes or until browned. Add red onion; cook and stir 3 minutes. Add garlic; cook and stir 1 minute more.

2. Add hominy to chicken mixture; cook and stir 4 minutes. Stir in chicken broth, olives, salsa, and bell pepper. Bring to boiling; reduce heat. Simmer, uncovered, about 10 minutes or until chicken is no longer pink. Remove from heat. Stir in cilantro.

3. If desired, top individual servings with avocado, sour cream, and cheese.

Nutrition facts per serving: 262 cal., 7 g total fat (1 g sat. fat), 44 mg chol., 933 mg sodium, 27 g carbo., 5 g fiber, 22 g pro.
Exchanges: ½ Vegetable, 1½ Starch, 2½ Very Lean Meat, 1 Fat

*Note: If you prefer spicy foods, use the greater amount of salsa.

For Wave 1, this is not appropriate. For Waves 2 and 3, serve with carrot sticks and fresh pineapple.

Olive Oil

Bell Peppers

WILD RICE CHICKEN SOUP

This easy-to make, hearty soup uses an abundance of tomatoes. Cooking them enhances their sweetness and activates their cancer-preventing properties

Prep: 30 minutes **Cook:** 40 minutes + 5 minutes **Makes:** 6 (1⅓-cup) servings

½ cup wild rice

2 cups water

½ cup long grain brown rice

2 14-ounce cans chicken broth

4 cloves garlic, minced (2 teaspoons minced)

4 cups chopped fresh tomatoes or two 14½-ounce cans diced tomatoes, undrained

2 cups chopped cooked chicken breast

1 cup finely chopped zucchini

¼ teaspoon freshly ground black pepper

1 tablespoon chopped fresh thyme

1 tablespoon Madeira or dry sherry (optional)

1. Rinse wild rice well; set aside. In a large saucepan bring the water to boiling. Add uncooked wild rice and brown rice. Return to boiling; reduce heat. Cover and simmer for 40 to 45 minutes or until rice is tender and most of the liquid is absorbed. Remove from heat; set aside.

2. Meanwhile, in a 4-quart Dutch oven combine chicken broth and garlic; bring to boiling. Stir in tomatoes, chicken, zucchini, and pepper. Return to boiling; reduce heat. Cover and simmer for 5 minutes. Stir in cooked rice, thyme, and, if desired, Madeira. Heat through.

Nutrition facts per serving: 218 cal., 3 g total fat (1 g sat. fat), 41 mg chol., 576 mg sodium, 29 g carbo., 3 g fiber, 20 g pro.
Exchanges: 1 Vegetable, 1½ Starch, 2 Very Lean Meat

For Wave 1, serve with Broccoli with Goat Cheese and Walnuts (page 211). For Waves 2 and 3, serve with fresh pear slices.

Whole Grains

Tomatoes

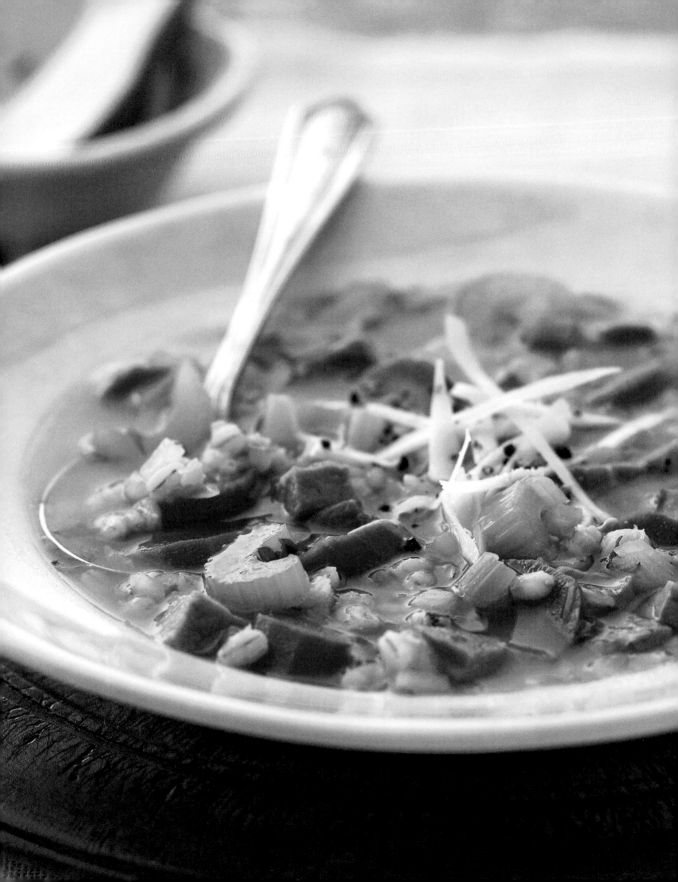

BARLEY MINESTRONE SOUP

Take time to savor this version of the Italian classic. A delightful blend of fresh herbs, vegetables, ham, and barley, this soup will satisfy your soul as well as your stomach.

Prep: 30 minutes **Cook:** 45 minutes **Makes:** 6 servings

2 tablespoons extra-virgin olive oil

2 cups chopped onion

6 cloves garlic, minced (1 tablespoon minced)

1 tablespoon chopped fresh rosemary

1 cup sliced celery

1 cup chopped cooked ham (about 5 ounces)

¾ cup regular barley (not quick-cooking), rinsed

8 cups reduced-sodium chicken broth or chicken stock

1½ cups sliced carrot

2 tablespoons chopped fresh flat-leaf parsley

2 teaspoons chopped fresh marjoram

2 teaspoons chopped fresh oregano

1 tablespoon lemon juice

2 tablespoons shredded Parmesan cheese

Cracked or freshly ground black pepper

1. In a 4- to 6-quart Dutch oven heat oil over medium heat. Add onion; cook until lightly golden brown, stirring occasionally. Add garlic and rosemary; cook and stir for 1 minute. Add celery, ham, and uncooked barley; cook for 4 minutes, stirring occasionally.

2. Add chicken broth. Bring to boiling; reduce heat. Cover and simmer for 30 minutes. Stir in carrot, parsley, marjoram, and oregano. Cover and simmer for 15 to 20 minutes more or until carrot and barley are tender.

3. Stir in lemon juice. Sprinkle individual servings with Parmesan cheese and cracked pepper.

Nutrition facts per serving: 212 cal., 6 g total fat (1 g sat. fat), 10 mg chol., 1,113 mg sodium, 29 g carbo., 6 g fiber, 12 g pro.
Exchanges: 1 Vegetable, 1½ Starch, 1 Lean Meat

For Wave 1, this is not appropriate. For Waves 2 and 3, serve with Stuffed Cherry Tomatoes (page 249) and fresh pear slices.

Olive Oil

Whole Grains

LENTIL AND ESCAROLE SOUP

Lentils are low in fat and high in protein and fiber; just look at how much fiber is in each bowl of this soup! Lentils, particularly the brown variety, cook quickly, so keep an eye on them or they will become mushy.

Prep: 35 minutes **Cook:** 20 minutes + 15 minutes **Makes:** 4 servings

1½ cups chopped onion

2 tablespoons extra-virgin olive oil

1 cup chopped carrot

6 cloves garlic, minced (1 tablespoon minced)

1 cup diced roma tomatoes

¾ cup dry brown lentils, rinsed and drained

6 cups water

10 cups torn fresh escarole or fresh spinach

2 tablespoons chopped fresh basil

1 tablespoon lemon juice (optional)

Kosher salt

Freshly ground black pepper

Extra-virgin olive oil, finely shredded Parmesan cheese, and/or chopped fresh flat-leaf parsley (optional)

1. In a 4- to 6-quart Dutch oven cook onion in the 2 tablespoons hot olive oil about 5 minutes or until tender, stirring occasionally. Add carrot and garlic; cook for 5 minutes more, stirring occasionally. Stir in tomatoes and lentils; cook and stir for 1 minute.

2. Add the water. Bring to boiling; reduce heat. Simmer, uncovered, for 20 minutes. Stir in escarole, if using. Simmer about 15 minutes more or until lentils are tender. Stir in spinach, if using.

3. Remove from heat. Stir in basil and, if desired, lemon juice. Season to taste with kosher salt and pepper. If desired, drizzle individual servings with olive oil and/or sprinkle with Parmesan cheese and/or parsley.

Nutrition facts per serving: 256 cal., 8 g total fat (1 g sat. fat), 0 mg chol., 124 mg sodium, 37 g carbo., 17 g fiber, 13 g pro.
Exchanges: 3 Vegetable, 1½ Starch, ½ Very Lean Meat, 1 Fat

For Wave 1, serve as is. For Waves 2 and 3, serve with fresh apple slices.

Olive Oil

Tomatoes

Spinach

SPICY BLACK BEAN CHILI

Don't be scared away by the seemingly long list of ingredients; many of them are seasonings you'll already have on hand. Black beans are great for cooking because they hold their shape; they also contain molybdenum, folate, fiber, and tryptophan.

Prep: 35 minutes **Cook:** 20 minutes **Makes:** 4 servings

2	tablespoons extra-virgin olive oil
1	tablespoon cumin seeds
2	cups chopped onion
½	cup chopped green bell pepper
2	cloves garlic, minced (1 teaspoon minced)
2	15-ounce cans black beans, rinsed and drained
1	14½-ounce can diced tomatoes, undrained
1½	cups water
1	tablespoon chili powder
2	teaspoons paprika
½	teaspoon crushed red pepper
1	tablespoon chopped fresh oregano
	Kosher salt
	Freshly ground black pepper
½	cup thinly sliced green onions
¼	cup fat-free dairy sour cream or plain low-fat yogurt
¼	cup chopped fresh cilantro

1. In a large saucepan heat olive oil over medium heat. Add the cumin seeds; cook and stir for 1 minute. Stir in chopped onion, bell pepper, and garlic. Cook and stir about 5 minutes or until onion is tender.

2. Stir in black beans, undrained tomatoes, the water, chili powder, paprika, and crushed red pepper.

3. Bring to boiling; reduce heat. Simmer, uncovered, for 20 minutes. Stir in oregano. Season to taste with kosher salt and black pepper.

4. Top individual servings with green onions, sour cream, and cilantro.

Nutrition facts per serving: 296 cal., 8 g total fat (1 g sat. fat), 3 mg chol., 799 mg sodium, 49 g carbo., 13 g fiber, 17 g pro.
Exchanges: 1½ Vegetable, 2 Starch, 1 Very Lean Meat, 1½ Fat

For Wave 1, serve with a mixed green salad. For Waves 2 and 3, serve with a whole grain roll and fresh mango slices.

Olive Oil   *Bell Peppers*

Tomatoes

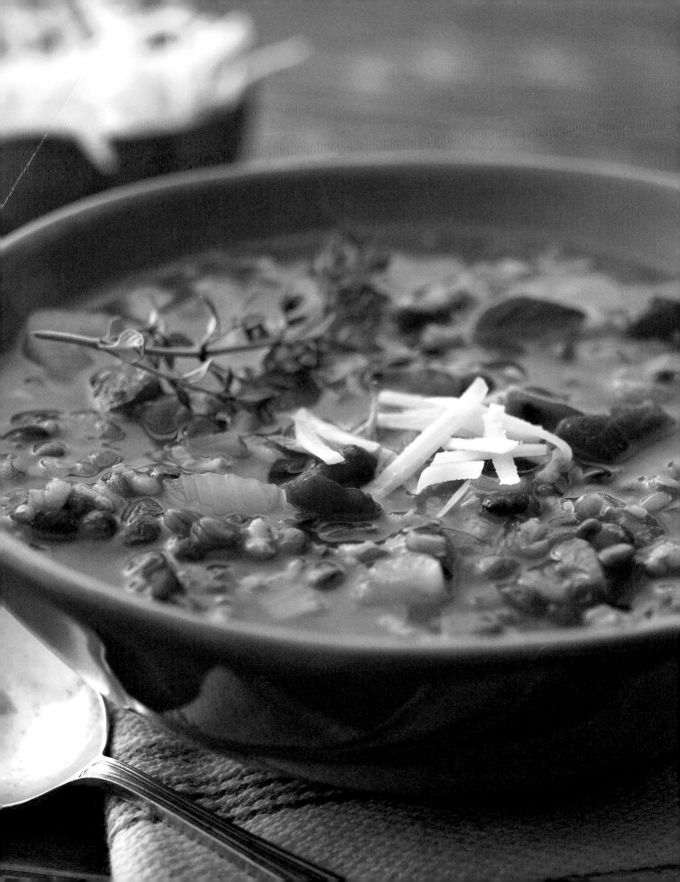

LENTIL SOUP WITH BROWN RICE

This warming soup is deliciously topped with a sprinkling of Asiago cheese.
Named after Asiago, Italy, the town where it was developed, it adds rich, nutty flavor.

Prep: 25 minutes **Cook:** 10 minutes + 30 minutes **Makes:** 6 servings

3 tablespoons extra-virgin olive oil

1 cup chopped onion

1 cup chopped celery

6 cloves garlic, minced (1 tablespoon minced)

8 cups reduced-sodium chicken broth or chicken stock

½ cup long grain brown rice

2 cups chopped tomato

¾ cup dry brown lentils, rinsed and drained

1 tablespoon chopped fresh thyme

1 tablespoon chopped fresh oregano

1 tablespoon lemon juice

¼ teaspoon freshly ground black pepper

2 tablespoons finely shredded Asiago cheese

Fresh thyme sprigs and/or oregano leaves

1. In a 4-quart Dutch oven heat olive oil over medium heat. Add onion, celery, and garlic; cook about 5 minutes or until tender, stirring occasionally. Stir in broth and uncooked brown rice. Bring to boiling; reduce heat. Simmer, uncovered, for 10 minutes. Stir in tomato and lentils. Return to boiling; reduce heat. Cover and simmer about 30 minutes more or until rice and lentils are tender.

2. Stir in thyme, oregano, lemon juice, and pepper. Top individual servings with Asiago cheese and, if desired, thyme sprigs and/or oregano leaves.

Nutrition facts per serving: 257 cal., 9 g total fat (2 g sat. fat), 3 mg chol., 810 mg sodium, 34 g carbo., 9 g fiber, 14 g pro.
Exchanges: ½ Vegetable, 2 Starch, 1 Very Lean Meat, 1½ Fat

For Wave 1, serve with Tomatoes with Crispy Bread Topping (page 207). For Waves 2 and 3, serve with Tomatoes with Crispy Bread Topping (page 207) and fresh grapes.

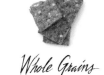

Olive Oil   *Tomatoes*

Whole Grains

TUSCAN TOMATO AND BREAD SOUP

This soup has such a rich, delicious base that you'll think it was made from cream. But it's really made from pureed tomatoes and vegetables. The bread makes a fun, crunchy topper.

Prep: 30 minutes **Bake:** 10 minutes **Cook:** 15 minutes + 15 minutes **Oven:** 350°F **Makes:** 6 servings

1 tablespoon extra-virgin olive oil

3 pounds fresh tomatoes, cored and coarsely chopped, or three 14½-ounce cans diced tomatoes, undrained

12 cloves garlic, minced (2 tablespoons minced)

¼ to ½ teaspoon crushed red pepper

2 14-ounce cans chicken broth

6 slices whole grain bread

1 tablespoon extra-virgin olive oil

4 cups chopped zucchini and/or yellow summer squash

2 tablespoons chopped fresh oregano

2 tablespoons chopped fresh flat-leaf parsley

Kosher salt

Freshly ground black pepper

1 ounce Parmesan cheese, shaved

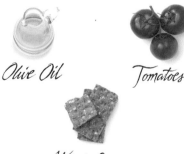

Olive Oil   *Tomatoes*

Whole Grains

1. In a 4-quart Dutch oven heat 1 tablespoon olive oil over medium heat. Reserve 1 cup of the chopped fresh tomatoes or, if using canned tomatoes, reserve 1 can of tomatoes. Add remaining fresh tomatoes or undrained canned tomatoes, the garlic, and crushed red pepper to hot oil in Dutch oven. Bring to boiling; reduce heat. Cover and cook for 15 to 20 minutes or until tomatoes are very tender, stirring occasionally. Add chicken broth. Bring to boiling; reduce heat. Cover and simmer for 15 minutes. Cool slightly.

2. Meanwhile, preheat oven to 350°F. Cut or tear bread into 1-inch pieces. Place in a shallow baking pan. Bake for 10 to 15 minutes or until toasted, stirring occasionally. Set aside. In a large skillet heat 1 tablespoon olive oil over medium heat. Add zucchini; cook for 3 to 5 minutes or until lightly browned and crisp-tender. Set aside.

3. Transfer half of the tomato and broth mixture to a blender or food processor. Cover and blend or process until smooth. Repeat with remaining half of the mixture. Return all to Dutch oven. If using canned tomatoes, drain the reserved can. Add reserved fresh or canned tomatoes, the cooked zucchini, the oregano, and parsley to pureed mixture. Season to taste with kosher salt and pepper. Heat through. Divide soup among six soup bowls. Top with bread pieces; garnish with cheese.

Nutrition facts per serving: 210 cal., 8 g total fat (2 g sat. fat), 5 mg chol., 796 mg sodium, 29 g carbo., 8 g fiber, 10 g pro.
Exchanges: 2 Vegetable, 1 Starch, 1½ Fat

For Wave 1, serve with low-fat cottage cheese. For Waves 2 and 3, serve with low-fat cottage cheese and fresh berries.

WHITE BEAN AND SQUASH STEW

The butternut squash in this hearty winter stew adds a touch of sweetness and tremendous flavor.
A topping of Manchego cheese melts beautifully and adds more intense golden color.

Prep: 30 minutes **Cook:** 15 minutes + 10 minutes **Makes:** 4 servings

1 tablespoon extra-virgin olive oil

2 cups chopped onion

6 cloves garlic, minced (1 tablespoon minced)

1 tablespoon sweet paprika

2 14-ounce cans chicken broth

3 cups 1-inch cubes peeled and seeded butternut squash

1 14½-ounce can diced tomatoes, undrained

1 tablespoon chopped fresh rosemary

1 19-ounce can cannellini beans (white kidney beans), rinsed and drained

2 tablespoons chopped fresh flat-leaf parsley

1 tablespoon chopped fresh thyme

Kosher salt

Freshly ground black pepper

2 tablespoons shaved Manchego cheese

1. In a large saucepan heat oil over medium heat. Add onion; cook about 5 minutes or until tender. Add garlic and paprika; cook for 2 minutes more. Add chicken broth, squash, undrained tomatoes, and rosemary. Bring to boiling; reduce heat. Cover and simmer about 15 minutes or until squash is tender.

2. Add beans, parsley, and thyme. Season to taste with kosher salt and pepper. Simmer, uncovered, for 10 minutes more.

3. Sprinkle individual servings with shaved Manchego cheese.

Nutrition facts per serving: 239 cal., 5 g total fat (1 g sat. fat), 4 mg chol., 1,376 mg sodium, 46 g carbo., 12 g fiber, 12 g pro.
Exchanges: 1 Vegetable, 2½ Starch, ½ Very Lean Meat, ½ Fat

For Wave 1, this is not appropriate. For Waves 2 and 3, serve with low-fat cottage cheese and fresh grapes.

Olive Oil

Tomatoes

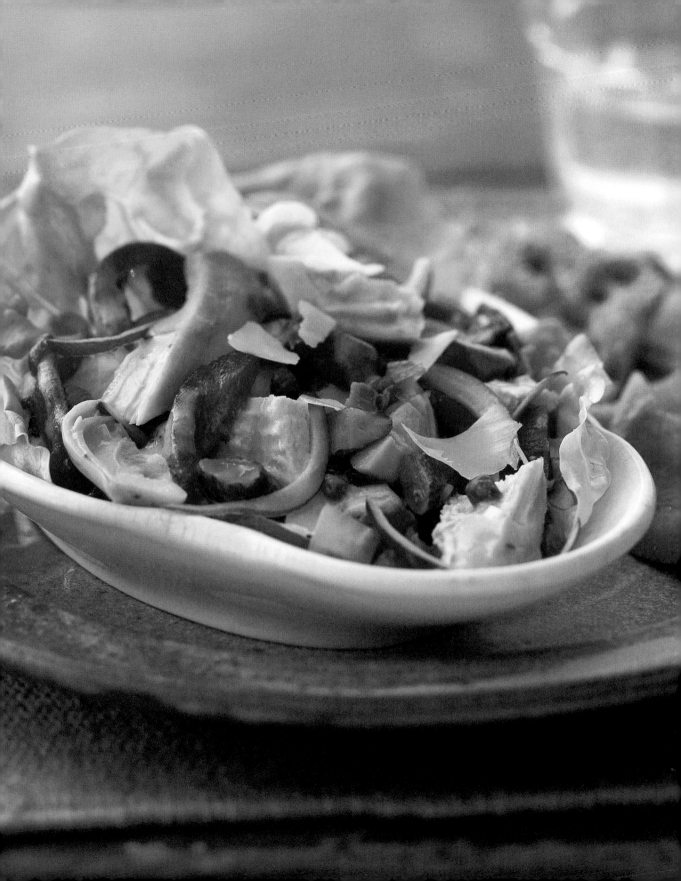

MEDITERRANEAN CHICKEN SALAD IN LETTUCE CUPS

Tender shredded chicken breasts and Mediterranean veggies marinated in a tangy red wine vinaigrette take on tremendous flavor. When served on top of a leaf of lettuce and sprinkled with Parmesan cheese, this simple salad becomes an elegant entrée.

Prep: 30 minutes   **Chill:** 1 to 24 hours   **Makes:** 6 servings

4   cups coarsely shredded cooked chicken breast (about 1¼ pounds)

1   15-ounce jar roasted red and yellow bell peppers, drained and cut into strips

1   6-ounce jar marinated artichoke hearts, drained and coarsely chopped

¼   cup thinly sliced red onion

¼   cup chopped almonds, toasted

2   tablespoons chopped fresh flat-leaf parsley

2   tablespoons capers, rinsed and drained

1   recipe Red Wine Vinaigrette

6   large butterhead (Bibb or Boston) lettuce leaves

2   ounces Parmesan cheese, shaved

1. In a large bowl combine chicken, roasted bell peppers, artichoke hearts, red onion, almonds, parsley, and capers. Drizzle with Red Wine Vinaigrette; toss gently to coat. Cover and chill for 1 to 24 hours.

2. To serve, place a lettuce leaf on each of six dinner plates. Spoon chicken salad onto lettuce leaves. Sprinkle with Parmesan cheese.

Nutrition facts per serving: 303 cal., 15 g total fat (3 g sat. fat), 86 mg chol., 466 mg sodium, 8 g carbo., 2 g fiber, 35 g pro.
Exchanges: 1½ Vegetable, 4½ Very Lean Meat, 2½ Fat

Red Wine Vinaigrette: In a small bowl combine 2 tablespoons red wine vinegar and 1 tablespoon finely chopped shallot. Let stand for 5 minutes. Whisk in 1½ teaspoons Dijon-style mustard. Add 2 tablespoons extra-virgin olive oil in a thin, steady stream, whisking constantly until combined. Stir in ⅛ teaspoon kosher salt and ⅛ teaspoon freshly ground black pepper. Makes about ⅓ cup.

For Wave 1, serve whole wheat pita wedges. For Waves 2 and 3, serve with whole wheat pita wedges and fresh apricot wedges.

Bell Peppers

Almonds

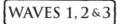 # CHICKEN-ORANGE SALAD

When time is of the essence, this speedy salad is just the meal you're looking for.
The handful of ingredients is ready to use, so all you have to do is toss them together.

Start to Finish: 15 minutes **Makes:** 4 servings

1   10-ounce package torn mixed salad greens

8   ounces cooked chicken breast, cut into
    bite-size pieces

⅓   cup bottled vinaigrette salad dressing
    (such as Newman's Own brand)

1   11-ounce can mandarin orange
    sections, drained

3   tablespoons sliced almonds, toasted

Almonds

1. In a large bowl combine greens and chicken.
Add salad dressing; toss to coat. Divide greens
mixture among four salad plates. Top with
mandarin orange sections and almonds.
Serve immediately.

Nutrition facts per serving: 230 cal., 11 g total fat
(2 g sat. fat), 48 mg chol., 289 mg sodium, 13 g carbo.,
2 g fiber, 20 g pro.
Exchanges: 2 Vegetable, ½ Fruit, 2½ Very Lean Meat,
1½ Fat

For Wave 1, do not top with the oranges.
Serve with a whole grain roll. For Waves 2 and
3, serve with a whole grain roll.

SONOMA *express* CHICKEN TOSSED SALAD

This combination of garlic-pepper chicken and vegetables offers another easy salad option when you're in a hurry or craving cool, fresh flavors.

Start to Finish: 20 minutes **Makes:** 4 servings

4 skinless, boneless chicken breast halves (about 1¼ pounds total)

1 tablespoon extra-virgin olive oil

¼ teaspoon garlic-pepper seasoning

8 cups torn mixed salad greens

1 medium yellow or red bell pepper, cut into bite-size strips

1 medium tomato, cut into wedges

½ cup bottled reduced-calorie berry or roasted garlic vinaigrette salad dressing

¼ cup crumbled feta cheese (1 ounce)

¼ cup whole wheat croutons (optional)

1. Brush chicken breasts with olive oil; sprinkle with garlic-pepper seasoning. In a large nonstick skillet cook chicken over medium heat for 8 to 10 minutes or until tender and no longer pink (170°F), turning once. Cut the chicken into bite-size strips. Set aside.

2. In a large serving bowl combine salad greens, bell pepper, and tomato. Pour salad dressing over greens mixture; toss gently to coat. Top with chicken, feta cheese, and, if desired, croutons.

Nutrition facts per serving: 312 cal., 10 g total fat (2 g sat. fat), 88 mg chol., 217 mg sodium, 20 g carbo., 2 g fiber, 36 g pro.
Exchanges: 2½ Vegetable, ½ Other Carbo., 4½ Very Lean Meat, 1½ Fat

For Wave 1, serve with toasted whole grain bread. For Waves 2 and 3, serve with toasted whole grain bread and fresh berries.

Olive Oil

Bell Peppers

Tomatoes

Whole Grains

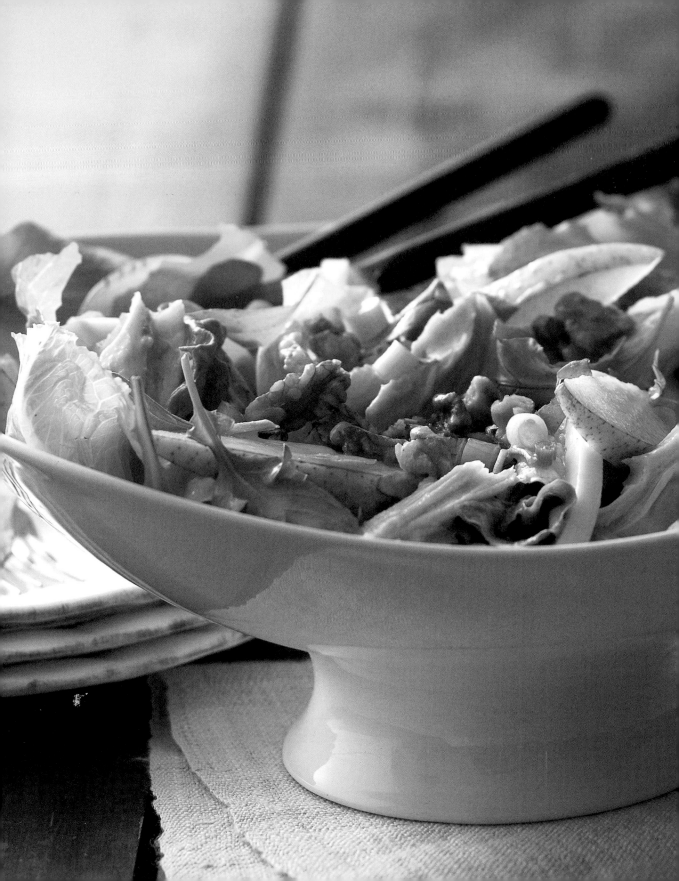

CHICKEN, PEAR, AND WALNUT SALAD

This lively salad is great for using up any leftover chicken you might have on hand and tempting enough that you'll gladly make a trip to the grocery store for more. Champagne vinegar lends mild delicacy to the dressing while Dijon mustard adds tang.

Start to Finish: 30 minutes **Makes:** 6 servings

12 ounces cooked chicken breast, shredded

 4 cups torn mixed greens

 4 cups torn arugula leaves

 4 ounces provolone cheese, cut into thin strips, or 2 ounces Gorgonzola cheese

 2 medium ripe pears, cored, halved, and thinly sliced

 2 tablespoons chopped fresh basil

 2 tablespoons chopped fresh mint

 ¼ cup Champagne vinegar

 2 tablespoons extra-virgin olive oil

 1 tablespoon Dijon-style mustard

 ⅔ cup chopped walnuts, toasted

 2 green onions, thinly sliced

1. In a very large bowl combine chicken, greens, arugula, cheese, pear slices, basil, and mint. Set aside.

2. In a screw-top jar combine Champagne vinegar, olive oil, and mustard. Cover and shake well. Drizzle over chicken mixture. Toss to coat. Top individual servings with walnuts and green onions.

Nutrition facts per serving: 336 cal., 21 g total fat (5 g sat. fat), 61 mg chol., 279 mg sodium, 13 g carbo., 4 g fiber, 26 g pro.
Exchanges: 1½ Vegetable, ½ Fruit, 2½ Very Lean Meat ½ High-Fat Meat, 3 Fat

For Wave 1, do not add the pears. Serve with a whole grain roll. For Waves 2 and 3, serve with a whole grain roll.

Olive Oil

SPINACH AND BASIL SALAD WITH BEEF

*Basil and spinach put a new spin on traditional iceberg- and romaine-based
salads while providing a vibrant backdrop for juicy fruits and beef.
A unique pear dressing makes this an elegant main-dish salad.*

Start to Finish: 25 minutes **Makes:** 2 main-dish servings

½ of a small very ripe pear, cored and peeled

1 tablespoon white wine vinegar or cider vinegar

¼ teaspoon Worcestershire sauce for chicken or regular Worcestershire sauce

Dash freshly ground black pepper

2 cups lightly packed torn fresh spinach

1 cup sliced fresh mushrooms

½ cup lightly packed fresh basil leaves

6 ounces sliced cooked beef, cut into thin strips (about 1 cup)

2 small oranges, peeled and sectioned, or one 11-ounce can mandarin orange sections, drained

2 tablespoons sliced almonds, toasted

1. For dressing, in a blender or food processor combine the pear, vinegar, Worcestershire sauce, and pepper. Cover and blend or process until smooth.

2. In a bowl toss together the spinach, mushrooms, and basil leaves. Add the beef strips and orange sections. Toss lightly to mix. Add the dressing; toss to mix. Sprinkle each serving with almonds to serve.

Nutrition facts per serving: 301 cal., 10 g total fat (2 g sat. fat), 75 mg chol., 67 mg sodium, 26 g carbo., 7 g fiber, 29 g pro.
Exchanges: 1½ Vegetable, 1½ Fruit, 3½ Lean Meat

For Wave 1, this is not appropriate. For Waves 2 and 3, serve with whole wheat pita wedges.

Almonds

Spinach

SONOMA *express* STEAK SALAD

*Likely to be a new favorite at your table, this vegetable and meat medley uses a delicious beef
and blue cheese duo for full, rich flavor on a foundation of soft, buttery Boston lettuce.*

Start to Finish: 25 minutes **Makes:** 4 main-dish servings

½ cup bottled red wine vinaigrette (such as Newman's Own)

1 tablespoon chopped fresh tarragon or ½ teaspoon dried tarragon, crushed

½ teaspoon cracked or coarsely ground black pepper

2 heads Boston lettuce, separated into leaves

8 ounces lean cooked beef, cut into thin bite-size strips

1 cup red or yellow baby pear tomatoes or cherry tomatoes

1 cup broccoli florets

½ of a medium red onion, cut into thin slices

¼ cup crumbled blue cheese (1 ounce)

½ cup whole wheat croutons

1. For dressing, combine salad dressing, tarragon, and pepper; set aside.

2. Line four dinner plates with lettuce leaves. Arrange beef, tomatoes, broccoli, and red onion on lettuce-lined plates. Sprinkle with blue cheese. Drizzle with dressing and top with croutons.

Nutrition facts per serving: 290 cal., 19 g total fat (4 g sat. fat), 55 mg chol., 496 mg sodium, 12 g carbo., 3 g fiber, 20 g pro.
Exchanges: 2½ Vegetable, 2 Lean Meat, 2½ Fat

For Wave 1, serve with whole wheat pita wedges. For Waves 2 and 3, serve with whole wheat pita wedges and fresh grapes.

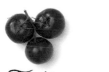

Tomatoes

Whole Grains

Broccoli

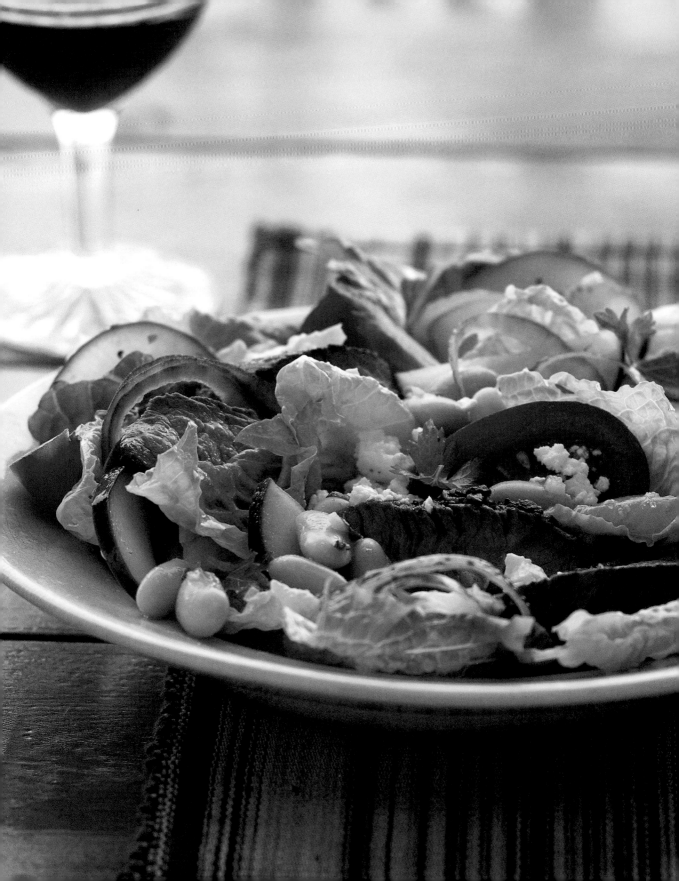

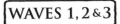

MEDITERRANEAN BEEF SALAD WITH LEMON VINAIGRETTE

A savory and zingy midday meal is the perfect rejuvenator on a long day. The contrasting textures and flavors of sirloin steak, fresh veggies, and crumbled feta complement each other and provide variety for your palate

Prep: 20 minutes **Broil:** 15 minutes **Makes:** 4 servings

1 pound boneless beef sirloin steak, cut 1 inch thick

Kosher salt

Freshly ground black pepper

4 cups torn romaine

1 small cucumber, sliced

½ of a small red onion, thinly sliced and separated into rings

1 cup halved cherry or grape tomatoes

1 cup canned cannellini beans (white kidney beans), rinsed and drained

½ cup crumbled feta cheese (2 ounces)

1 recipe Lemon Vinaigrette

Fresh flat-leaf parsley (optional)

Tomatoes

1. Preheat broiler. Trim fat from steak. Season steak with kosher salt and pepper. Place steak on the unheated rack of a broiler pan. Broil 3 to 4 inches from the heat until desired doneness, turning once. Allow 15 to 17 minutes for medium-rare doneness (145°F) or 20 to 22 minutes for medium doneness (160°F.) Thinly slice the meat.

2. Divide torn romaine among four dinner plates. Top with sliced meat, cucumber slices, red onion, tomatoes, cannellini beans, and feta cheese. Drizzle with Lemon Vinaigrette. If desired, garnish with parsley.

Nutrition facts per serving: 370 cal., 21 g total fat (5 g sat. fat), 81 mg chol., 514 mg sodium, 18 g carbo., 6 g fiber, 32 g pro.
Exchanges: 2 Vegetable, ½ Starch, 4 Very Lean Meat, 1½ Fat

Lemon Vinaigrette: In a screw-top jar combine ¼ cup extra-virgin olive oil, ½ teaspoon finely shredded lemon peel, 3 tablespoons lemon juice, 1 tablespoon chopped fresh oregano, and 2 cloves garlic, minced (1 teaspoon minced). Cover and shake well. Season to taste with kosher salt and freshly ground black pepper. Makes about ½ cup.

For Wave 1, serve as is. For Waves 2 and 3, serve with fresh peach slices.

CURRIED CHICKEN WRAPS

Curry, coriander, and mango combine in this wrap to bring you a taste of the exotic. Chicken may be the meat of the dish, but mango steals the show with its vibrant orange color, amazing aroma, and sweet-tart flavor.

Prep: 25 minutes **Marinate:** 30 minutes **Makes:** 6 servings

12 ounces skinless, boneless chicken breast halves, cut into ¼-inch-thick slices

1 tablespoon extra-virgin olive oil

1 tablespoon curry powder

1 teaspoon ground coriander

½ teaspoon kosher salt

¼ teaspoon freshly ground black pepper

1 tablespoon extra-virgin olive oil

1 cup thinly sliced red onion

1 cup chopped mango

2 cups shredded romaine

1 cup watercress, tough stems removed

2 tablespoons lemon juice

2 teaspoons extra-virgin olive oil

6 7- to 8-inch whole wheat flour tortillas

1. In a medium bowl combine chicken, 1 tablespoon olive oil, curry powder, coriander, kosher salt, and pepper. Cover and marinate in the refrigerator for 30 minutes.

2. In a large skillet heat 1 tablespoon olive oil over medium heat. Add the chicken and red onion; cook and stir for 4 to 6 minutes or until chicken is tender and no longer pink. Add mango; cook and stir until heated through.

3. Meanwhile, in a medium bowl combine romaine and watercress. Drizzle with lemon juice and the 2 teaspoons olive oil; toss gently to coat.

4. To serve, divide the chicken mixture and romaine mixture among tortillas. Roll up tortillas.

Nutrition facts per serving: 291 cal., 10 g total fat (2 g sat. fat), 33 mg chol., 576 mg sodium, 35 g carbo., 4 g fiber, 18 g pro.
Exchanges: 1 Vegetable, 1½ Starch, 2 Very Lean Meat, 1½ Fat

For Wave 1, do not add the mango. Serve with cucumber slices. For Waves 2 and 3, serve with kiwifruit.

Olive Oil

Whole Grains

TURKEY-APPLE SALAD WRAPS

If finger foods aren't your style, skip the wrapping step of this recipe and simply serve the sweet and savory turkey mixture over lettuce.

Start to Finish: 30 minutes **Makes:** 4 servings

12 ounces cooked turkey breast, shredded

1 cup chopped green apple

½ cup chopped celery

½ cup chopped walnuts, toasted

½ cup sliced green onions

½ cup chopped fresh flat-leaf parsley

¼ cup dried tart cherries

½ cup light dairy sour cream

2 tablespoons lemon juice

½ to 1 teaspoon bottled hot pepper sauce

¼ teaspoon kosher salt

¼ teaspoon freshly ground black pepper

12 butterhead (Boston or Bibb) lettuce leaves

1. In a large bowl combine the turkey, apple, celery, walnuts, green onions, parsley, and cherries.

2. In a small bowl stir together the sour cream, lemon juice, hot pepper sauce, kosher salt, and black pepper. Add the sour cream mixture to the turkey mixture, stir until well mixed.

3. Divide turkey mixture among lettuce leaves, spooning turkey mixture into center of each leaf.° Fold bottom edge of each lettuce leaf up and over filling. Fold opposite sides in and over filling. Roll up from the bottom.

Nutrition facts per serving: 313 cal., 13 g total fat (3 g sat. fat), 81 mg chol., 205 mg sodium, 19 g carbo., 4 g fiber, 31 g pro.
Exchanges: 1½ Vegetable, ½ Fruit, 4 Very Lean Meat, 2 Fat

*****Note:** If you prefer, serve the turkey mixture over torn lettuce.

For Wave 1, this is not appropriate. For Waves 2 and 3, serve with whole wheat pita wedges and apple slices.

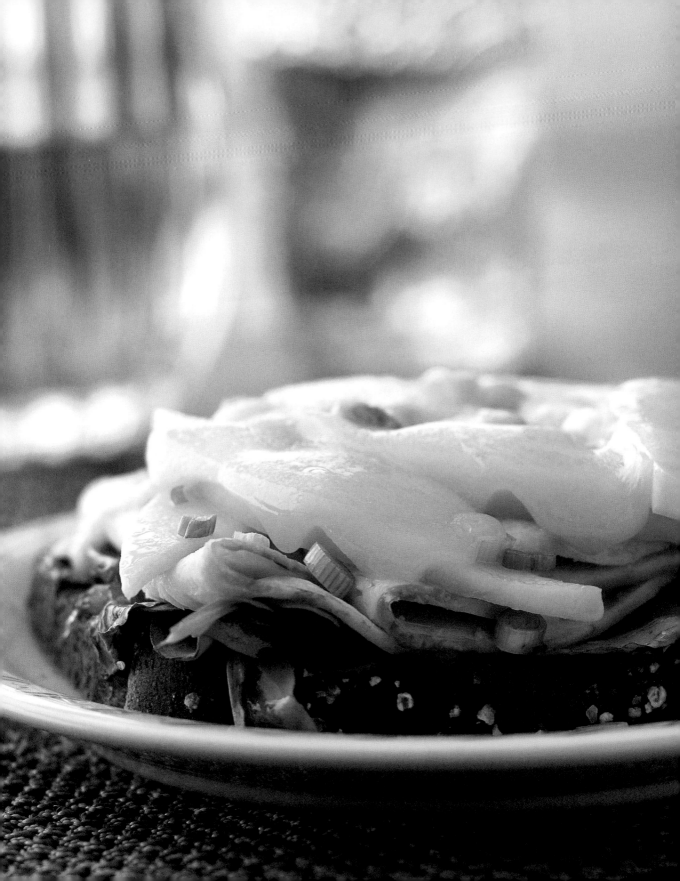

TURKEY MANGO MELTS

*This warm, cheesy melt is simple and speedy and still full of nutrients.
Fresh mango alone contains vitamins A, C, and D.*

Start to Finish: 15 minutes **Makes:** 4 servings

4 slices whole wheat bread

2 tablespoons mango chutney

2 cups arugula leaves

6 ounces thinly sliced cooked turkey breast

1 large mango, seeded, peeled, and sliced

2 tablespoons sliced green onion

4 1-ounce slices Swiss cheese

Whole Grains

1. Preheat broiler. Arrange bread on the unheated rack of a broiler pan. Snip any large pieces of fruit in the chutney. Spread top of each bread slice with one-quarter of the mango chutney. Top with arugula, turkey, mango slices, and green onion. Add Swiss cheese.

2. Broil 3 to 4 inches from the heat about 2 minutes or until cheese begins to melt. Serve immediately.

Nutrition facts per serving: 255 cal., 9 g total fat
(5 g sat. fat), 41 mg chol., 675 mg sodium, 26 g carbo.,
3 g fiber, 19 g pro.
Exchanges: ½ Fruit, 1 Starch, ½ Other Carbo.,
2 Very Lean Meat, 1 Fat

*For Wave 1, this is not appropriate. For Waves
2 and 3, serve with additional fresh mango slices
and bell pepper strips.*

TUSCAN-STYLE EGGPLANT SANDWICHES

Tuscan cuisine is appreciated throughout the world for its natural and flavorful ingredients and dishes that are wholesome, tasty, and simple. Keeping true to Tuscan tradition, this recipe has only a few basic ingredients, all full of flavor.

Prep: 20 minutes **Bake:** 15 minutes **Cook:** 6 minutes per batch **Oven:** 350°F **Makes:** 4 servings

2   medium eggplant (2 to 2½ pounds total)

¼   cup extra-virgin olive oil

½   teaspoon kosher salt

½   teaspoon freshly ground black pepper

¼   cup dried tomatoes (not oil-packed)

1½ cups shredded part-skim mozzarella cheese (6 ounces)

2   tablespoons chopped fresh basil

1   cup purchased tomato pasta sauce, warmed

Olive Oil

Tomatoes

1. Preheat oven to 350°F. Trim ends off eggplant and discard. Cut eggplant crosswise into ½-inch-thick slices (16 to 20 slices total). Arrange slices in a single layer on a large baking sheet. Brush eggplant with 2 tablespoons of the olive oil; sprinkle with the kosher salt and pepper. Bake about 15 minutes or until eggplant is tender. Let cool on baking sheet on a wire rack.

2. Meanwhile, place dried tomatoes in a small bowl; add enough boiling water to cover. Let stand for 10 minutes. Drain tomatoes and squeeze out any excess water. Finely chop tomatoes and set aside.

3. Divide the cheese among half of the eggplant slices, leaving a ⅛-inch border around the edges of the slices. Sprinkle dried tomatoes and basil evenly over cheese. Top with remaining eggplant slices, pressing down to compact slightly.

4. In a large nonstick skillet heat 1 tablespoon of the remaining olive oil over medium heat. Add half of the eggplant stacks. Cook for 6 to 8 minutes or until browned and cheese is melted, turning once halfway through cooking. Remove eggplant stacks from skillet; cover to keep warm. Repeat with remaining 1 tablespoon olive oil and remaining eggplant stacks.

5. Serve eggplant stacks with warmed pasta sauce.

Nutrition facts per serving: 332 cal., 22 g total fat (7 g sat. fat), 27 mg chol., 775 mg sodium, 22 g carbo., 9 g fiber, 14 g pro.
Exchanges: 3 Vegetable, ½ Other Carbo., 1½ Very Lean Meat, 3½ Fat

For Wave 1, serve with whole wheat pita wedges. For Waves 2 and 3, serve with whole wheat pita wedges and fresh nectarine slices.

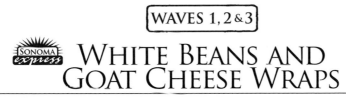

WHITE BEANS AND GOAT CHEESE WRAPS

Goat cheese has a surprisingly tart flavor that contrasts the mild flavor of cannellini beans and works in tandem with the sweetness of the roasted red peppers to create a flavor-packed wrap.

Start to Finish: 20 minutes **Makes:** 6 servings

1   19-ounce can cannellini beans (white kidney beans), rinsed and drained

1   4-ounce package soft goat cheese (chèvre)

1   tablespoon chopped fresh oregano

1   tablespoon chopped fresh flat-leaf parsley

6   8-inch whole wheat flour tortillas, warmed* if desired

6   cups fresh baby spinach leaves

1   12-ounce jar roasted red bell peppers, drained and thinly sliced

1. In a medium bowl mash beans lightly with a fork. Add goat cheese, oregano, and parsley; stir until well mixed.

2. Divide bean mixture among tortillas, spreading evenly. Top bean mixture with spinach and roasted peppers. Roll up tortillas; cut in half to serve.

Nutrition facts per serving: 218 cal., 8 g total fat (4 g sat. fat), 9 mg chol., 552 mg sodium, 31 g carbo., 16 g fiber, 18 g pro.
Exchanges: 1½ Vegetable, 1½ Starch, 1 Very Lean Meat, ½ Medium-Fat Meat, ½ Fat

*Note: To warm tortillas, preheat oven to 350°F. Wrap tortillas tightly in foil. Bake about 10 minutes or until heated through.

For Wave 1, serve as is. For Waves 2 and 3, serve with fresh berries.

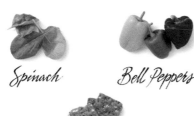

Spinach   *Bell Peppers*

Whole Grains

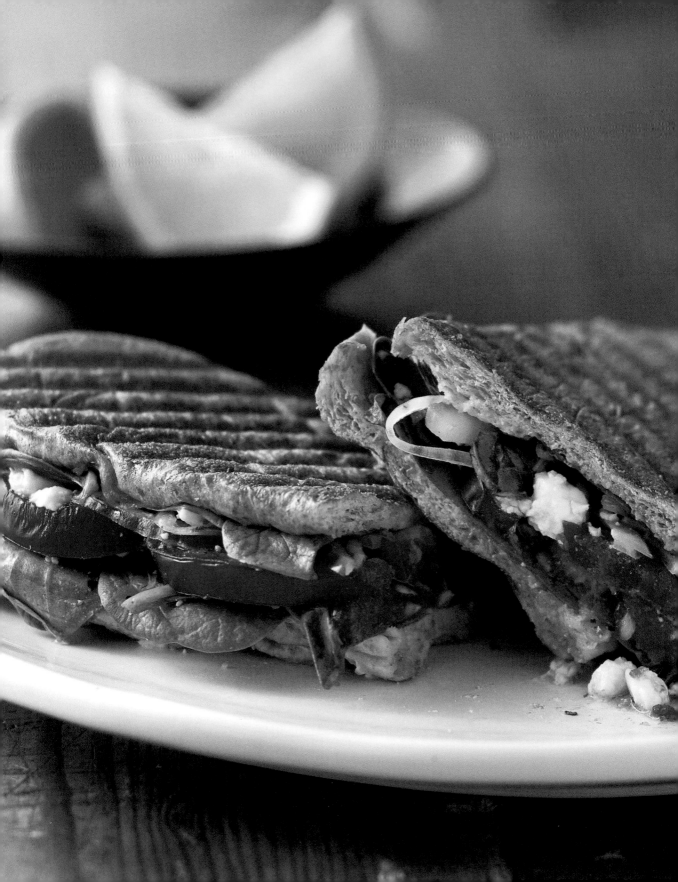

![Sonoma express] SPINACH PANINI

With half of its ingredients on the list of Sonoma Power Foods, this grilled Italian sandwich packs a nutritional punch. Spinach is rich in carotenoids, folate, vitamin K, and magnesium.

Prep: 20 minutes **Cook:** 2 minutes per batch **Makes:** 4 servings

Nonstick olive oil cooking spray

4 6-inch whole wheat hoagie rolls, split; 8 slices whole wheat bread; or 2 whole wheat pita bread rounds, halved crosswise and split horizontally

4 cups fresh baby spinach leaves

8 thin tomato slices (1 medium tomato)

¼ teaspoon kosher salt

⅛ teaspoon freshly ground black pepper

¼ cup thinly sliced red onion

2 tablespoons shredded fresh basil leaves

½ cup crumbled feta cheese (2 ounces)

Olive Oil

Spinach

Tomatoes

Whole Grains

1. Lightly coat an unheated panini griddle, covered indoor electric grill, or large nonstick skillet with nonstick cooking spray; set aside.

2. Place hoagie roll bottoms or 4 of the bread slices or 4 pita pieces on a work surface; divide half of the spinach leaves among these roll bottoms, bread slices, or pita pieces. Top spinach with tomato and sprinkle lightly with kosher salt and pepper. Add red onion slices and basil. Top with feta and remaining spinach. Top with hoagie roll tops, remaining bread slices, or pita pieces. Press down firmly.

3. Preheat griddle, grill, or skillet over medium heat or heat according to manufacturer's directions. Add sandwiches, in batches if necessary. If using griddle or grill, close lid and grill for 2 to 3 minutes or until bread is toasted. (If using skillet, place a heavy plate on top of sandwiches. Cook for 1 to 2 minutes or until bottoms are toasted. Carefully remove plate, which may be hot. Turn sandwiches and top with the plate. Cook for 1 to 2 minutes more or until bread is toasted.)

Nutrition facts per serving: 299 cal., 7 g total fat (3 g sat. fat), 13 mg chol., 826 mg sodium, 50 g carbo., 8 g fiber, 13 g pro.
Exchanges: 1½ Vegetable, 3 Starch, ½ Medium-Fat Meat

For Wave 1, serve as is. For Waves 2 and 3, serve with fresh orange slices.

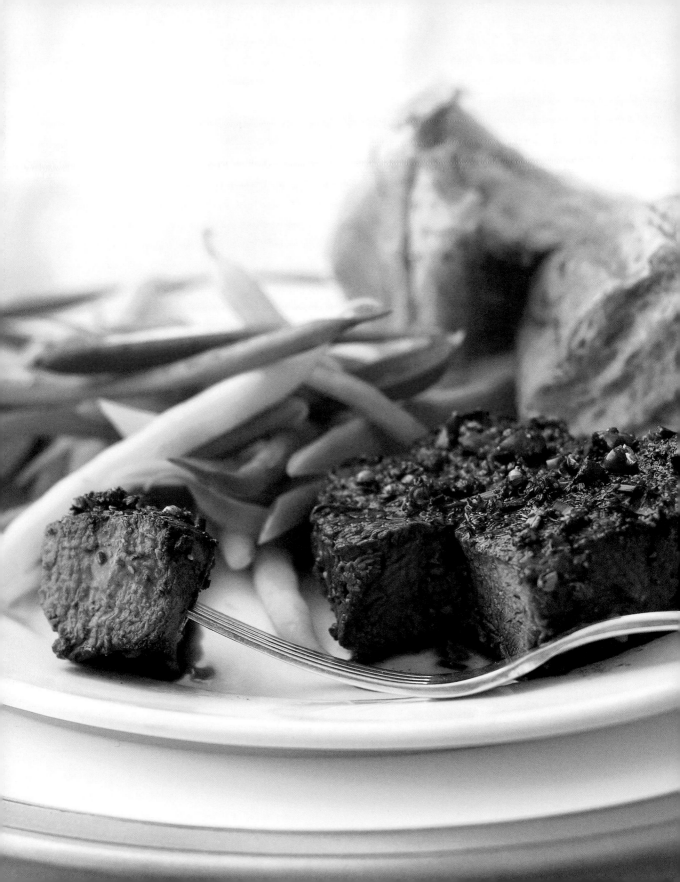

Beef Entrées

Lean cuts of beef fill your Sonoma Diet protein needs perfectly. Here you'll find a world of ideas for making this old favorite new again. From Japanese-style teriyaki beef spirals to South American flank steak, from Thai roast beef to the chipotle skirt steaks of Mexico, far-flung flavors will turn your kitchen into a fiesta. But remember, though the tastes are far reaching, the ingredients are as close as your neighborhood supermarket.

PEPPERED BEEF WITH WATERCRESS

This stylish steak dish is loaded with more than just tremendous flavor. The watercress contributes antioxidants, phytochemicals, iron, and vitamins A and C while lending additional peppery flavor.

Prep: 20 minutes **Cook:** 12 minutes **Makes:** 4 servings

1 pound boneless beef flatiron or ribeye steak, cut about 1 inch thick

2 tablespoons freshly ground black pepper

1 tablespoon fennel seeds, crushed

½ teaspoon kosher salt

Nonstick cooking spray

2 cups watercress, tough stems removed

2 cups thinly sliced celery

1 cup sliced, seeded cucumber

½ cup shelled fresh or frozen sweet soybeans (edamame), thawed if necessary, or canned cannellini beans, rinsed and drained (optional)

3 tablespoons extra-virgin olive oil

2 tablespoons lemon juice

1 tablespoon chopped fresh chives

Olive Oil

1. Trim fat from meat. Cut meat into 4 portions. Season meat evenly with pepper, fennel seeds, and kosher salt; rub in with your fingers. Set aside.

2. Lightly coat an unheated large skillet with nonstick cooking spray. Preheat skillet over medium-high heat. Add meat. Reduce heat to medium; cook for 12 to 15 minutes or until desired doneness (145°F for medium-rare doneness or 160°F for medium doneness), turning meat occasionally to brown evenly. (If meat browns too quickly, reduce heat to medium-low.)

3. Meanwhile, in a large bowl combine watercress, celery, cucumber, sweet soybeans (if using), olive oil, lemon juice, and chives; toss to combine. Divide watercress mixture among four dinner plates. Top each serving with one portion meat.

Nutrition facts per serving: 296 cal., 19 g total fat (5 g sat. fat), 66 mg chol., 360 mg sodium, 6 g carbo., 3 g fiber, 24 g pro.
Exchanges: ½ Other Carbo., 3 Lean Meat, 2 Fat

For Wave 1, serve with Wild Rice Stuffing (page 257). For Waves 2 and 3, serve with Wild Rice Stuffing (page 257) and fresh apple slices.

Wine Pairing: Cabernet Sauvignon

SICILIAN-STYLE BEEF STEAK

The island of Sicily boasts some of Italy's most elegant and delicious dishes.
You can enjoy this Sicilian-style meal from your own kitchen. Italian flat-leaf parsley is
used as more than a simple garnish here; it adds color, flavor, and vitamins A and C.

Start to Finish: 40 minutes **Makes:** 4 servings

1 pound boneless beef sirloin steak,
   cut 1 inch thick

½ teaspoon kosher salt

¼ teaspoon freshly ground black pepper

2 tablespoons extra-virgin olive oil

½ cup finely chopped celery

1 14-ounce can whole tomatoes,
   undrained, cut up

¾ cup sliced pitted ripe olives

1 tablespoon capers, rinsed and drained

2 teaspoons chopped fresh oregano

1 clove garlic, minced (½ teaspoon minced)

¼ teaspoon crushed red pepper

2 tablespoons chopped fresh
   flat-leaf parsley

1. Trim fat from meat. Season meat with kosher salt and black pepper.

2. In a large skillet cook heat olive oil over medium heat. Add meat; cook for 8 to 10 minutes or until browned, turning once. Remove meat from skillet.

3. In the same skillet cook celery over medium-low heat about 4 minutes or just until tender. Stir in undrained tomatoes, olives, capers, oregano, garlic, and crushed red pepper. Bring to boiling; reduce heat. Simmer, uncovered, until liquid begins to thicken. Return meat and any accumulated juices to the skillet. Simmer, uncovered, for 5 to 10 minutes or until meat is desired doneness (145°F for medium-rare doneness or 160°F for medium doneness).

4. To serve, remove meat from tomato mixture; cut into thin slices. Stir parsley into tomato mixture in skillet; serve over meat.

Nutrition facts per serving: 262 cal., 15 g total fat (3 g sat. fat), 69 mg chol., 721 mg sodium, 7 g carbo., 2 g fiber, 25 g pro.
Exchanges: 1 Vegetable, 3½ Very Lean Meat, 1 Fat

For Wave 1, serve with cooked multigrain pasta and cooked broccoli. For Waves 2 and 3, serve with cooked multigrain pasta, cooked broccoli, and fresh grapes.

Wine Pairing: Zinfandel

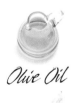

Olive Oil

Tomatoes

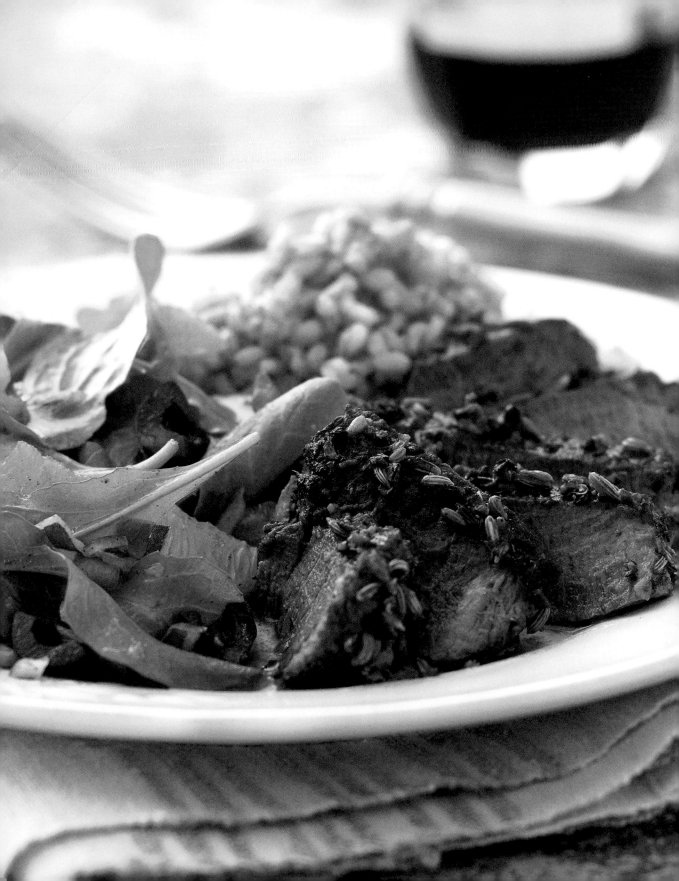

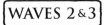
SEARED BEEF WITH ORANGE SALSA

Searing beef is a convenient cooking method that takes only minutes and seals in the meat's juices to ensure a tender steak. This recipe has a distinct citrus twist from the inclusion of oranges and lemon juice.

Start to Finish: 35 minutes **Makes:** 4 servings

4   large oranges

2   teaspoons fennel seeds, crushed

2   teaspoons black peppercorns, crushed

¼   teaspoon kosher salt

12 ounces beef tenderloin, cut into 4 steaks (each about ¾ inch thick)

1   tablespoon extra-virgin olive oil

½   cup finely chopped red onion

¼   cup pitted kalamata olives, quartered

¼   cup chopped fresh flat-leaf parsley

2   tablespoons lemon juice

2   tablespoons extra-virgin olive oil

1   clove garlic, minced (½ teaspoon minced)

½   teaspoon paprika

4   cups torn arugula leaves

Olive Oil

1. Finely shred enough of the orange peel to make 2 teaspoons. In a small bowl combine orange peel, fennel seeds, peppercorns, and kosher salt. Sprinkle mixture evenly over beef.

2. In a large skillet heat the 1 tablespoon olive oil over medium-high heat; add the meat. Reduce heat to medium. Cook for 7 to 9 minutes or until desired doneness (145°F for medium rare doneness or 160°F for medium doneness), turning once. Slice meat across the grain into thin slices.

3. Meanwhile, peel oranges, removing all of the white pith. Section oranges. In a large bowl combine orange sections, red onion, olives, parsley, lemon juice, the 2 tablespoons olive oil, the garlic, and paprika. Stir gently to combine.

4. Add arugula to orange mixture; toss to combine. Divide arugula mixture among four dinner plates. Serve with sliced meat.

Nutrition facts per serving: 318 cal., 18 g total fat (4 g sat. fat), 52 mg chol., 263 mg sodium, 21 g carbo., 5 g fiber, 20 g pro.
Exchanges: 1 Vegetable, 1 Fruit, 2½ Lean Meat, 2 Fat

For Wave 1, this is not appropriate. For Waves 2 and 3, serve with cooked brown rice.

Wine Suggestion: Sparkling semisweet or rosé

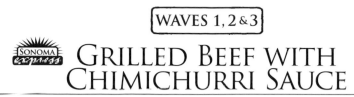

GRILLED BEEF WITH CHIMICHURRI SAUCE

A traditional sauce of Argentina, chimichurri is loaded with fresh herbs and seasonings. It's used in Argentina the way Americans use ketchup and is a must on grilled meat, particularly beef.

Prep: 15 minutes **Grill:** 12 minutes **Makes:** 4 servings

¼   cup chopped fresh flat-leaf parsley

2   tablespoons red wine vinegar

2   tablespoons extra-virgin olive oil

2   tablespoons beef broth or water

2   tablespoons finely chopped shallot

1   tablespoon chopped fresh oregano

4   cloves garlic, minced (2 teaspoons minced)

½   teaspoon lemon juice

¼   teaspoon crushed red pepper

    Kosher salt

1   1-pound beef flank steak

    Freshly ground black pepper

Olive Oil

1. For chimichurri sauce, in a small bowl combine parsley, red wine vinegar, olive oil, broth, shallot, oregano, garlic, lemon juice, and crushed red pepper. Season to taste with kosher salt. Cover and let stand at room temperature for 1 hour. (Or prepare sauce; cover and chill in the refrigerator for up to 48 hours. Let stand at room temperature before using.)

2. Trim fat from steak. Score both sides of steak in a diamond pattern by making shallow diagonal cuts at 1-inch intervals. Season meat with kosher salt and black pepper. For a charcoal grill, place steak on the rack of an uncovered grill directly over medium coals. Grill for 12 to 14 minutes or until medium doneness (160°F). (For a gas grill, preheat grill. Reduce heat to medium. Place steak on grill rack over heat. Cover and grill as above.) Serve steak with chimichurri sauce.

Nutrition facts per serving: 236 cal., 13 g total fat (4 g sat. fat), 47 mg chol., 207 mg sodium, 2 g carbo., 0 g fiber, 25 g pro.
Exchanges: 3½ Lean Meat, 1 Fat

For Wave 1, serve with whole grain bread and cooked red bell peppers with green beans. For Waves 2 and 3, serve with whole grain bread, cooked red bell peppers with green beans, and fresh orange slices.

Wine Pairing: Pinot Noir

GRILLED FIVE-SPICE FLANK STEAK

The combination of Japanese and Chinese ingredients gives this Asian-inspired dish exceptional flavor. The small amount of mirin lends a rich aroma and sweetness. The alcohol content of mirin, although low, makes it easier for ingredients to absorb flavors, so you don't need a long marinating time.

Prep: 15 minutes   **Marinate:** 30 minutes to 4 hours   **Grill:** 17 minutes   **Makes:** 4 servings

1   1-pound beef flank steak

Kosher salt

Freshly ground black pepper

2   tablespoons soy sauce

1   tablespoon sweet rice wine (mirin)

1   tablespoon lemon juice

4   cloves garlic, minced (2 teaspoons minced)

2   teaspoons grated fresh ginger

2   teaspoons five-spice powder

2   teaspoons ground coriander

1   teaspoon toasted sesame oil

¼   teaspoon fennel seeds, crushed

Dash cayenne pepper

1. Trim fat from steak. Season steak with kosher salt and black pepper. Place steak in a large self-sealing plastic bag set in a shallow dish.

2. For marinade, in a small bowl combine soy sauce, sweet rice wine, lemon juice, garlic, ginger, five-spice powder, coriander, sesame oil, fennel seeds, and cayenne pepper. Pour marinade over steak. Seal bag; turn to coat steak. Marinate in the refrigerator for 30 minutes to 4 hours, turning bag occasionally.

3. Drain steak, discarding marinade. For a charcoal grill, place steak on the rack of an uncovered grill directly over medium coals. Grill for 17 to 21 minutes or until medium doneness (160°F), turning once halfway through grilling. (For a gas grill, preheat grill. Reduce heat to medium. Place steak on grill rack over heat. Cover and grill as above.)

4. To serve, thinly slice steak across the grain.

Nutrition facts per serving: 204 cal., 8 g total fat (3 g sat. fat), 47 mg chol., 689 mg sodium, 6 g carbo., 1 g fiber, 26 g pro.
Exchanges: 3½ Lean Meat

Note: This marinade can be used on other cuts of meat, such as beef tenderloin, New York strip steak, pork tenderloin, or chicken breast halves.

For Wave 1, serve with Mushrooms with Garlic and Herbs (page 209), steamed bell peppers with eggplant, and cooked multigrain pasta. For Waves 2 and 3, serve with Shaved Fennel with Oranges and Pomegranates (page 252) and cooked multigrain pasta.

Wine Pairing: Merlot

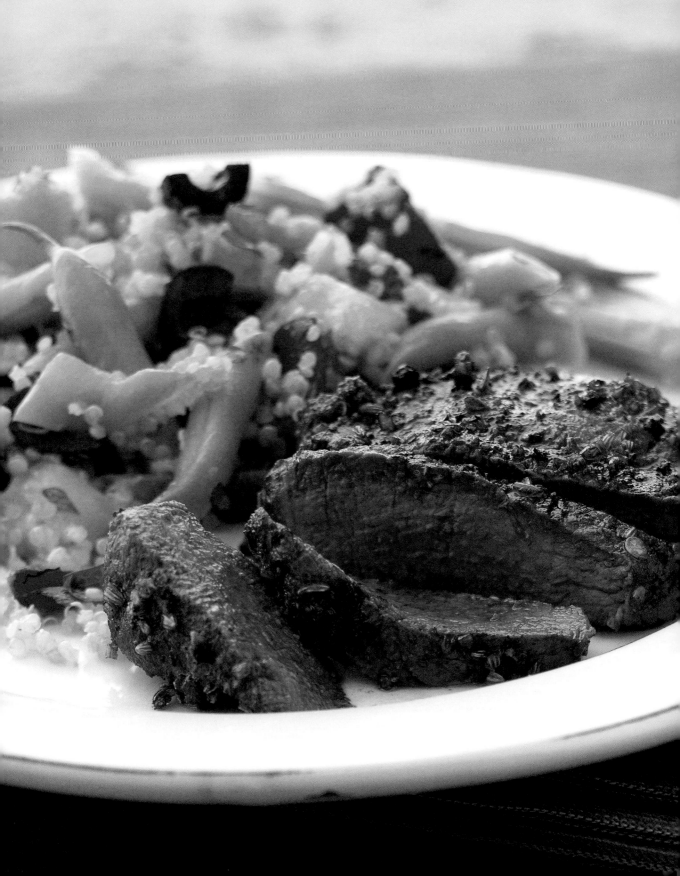

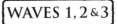
GRILLED BEEF WITH QUINOA AND VEGETABLES

Although quinoa is filling the grain portion of your plate, it is also a complete protein source because it contains all eight essential amino acids. Its unique texture and delicate flavor perfectly complement this meaty meal.

Prep: 30 minutes **Grill:** 10 minutes **Makes:** 4 servings

1 cup water

½ cup quinoa*

2 cups fresh green beans, bias-sliced into 2-inch pieces

4 beef tenderloin steaks, cut 1 inch thick (about 1 pound total)

2 tablespoons extra-virgin olive oil

1 tablespoon fennel seeds, crushed

Kosher salt

Freshly ground black pepper

1 cup bottled roasted red and/or yellow bell peppers, drained and chopped

2 tablespoons red wine vinegar

1 tablespoon chopped pitted kalamata olives

2 teaspoons chopped fresh flat-leaf parsley

1. In a medium saucepan bring the water to boiling. Add quinoa and return to boiling; reduce heat. Cover and simmer about 15 minutes or until quinoa is tender and most of the liquid is absorbed. Remove from heat; set aside.

2. Meanwhile, in a covered medium saucepan cook green beans in a small amount of lightly salted boiling water for 5 minutes. Drain; submerse green beans in ice water to stop the cooking process. Drain well.

3. Meanwhile, drizzle the steaks with 1 tablespoon of the olive oil. Sprinkle with crushed fennel seeds; season meat with kosher salt and black pepper.

4. For a charcoal grill, place steaks on the rack of an uncovered grill directly over medium coals. Grill 10 to 12 minutes for medium-rare doneness (145°F) or 12 to 15 minutes for medium doneness (160°F), turning once halfway through grilling. (For a gas grill, preheat grill. Reduce heat to medium. Place steaks on grill rack over heat. Cover and grill as above.)

5. In a large bowl combine cooked quinoa, green beans, roasted peppers, red wine vinegar, olives, parsley, and the remaining 1 tablespoon olive oil. Season to taste with kosher salt and black pepper.

6. To serve, divide quinoa mixture among four dinner plates. Top with the steaks.

Nutrition facts per serving: 351 cal., 17 g total fat (4 g sat. fat), 70 mg chol., 208 mg sodium, 22 g carbo., 5 g fiber, 28 g pro.
Exchanges: 1 Vegetable, 1 Starch, 3 Lean Meat, 2 Fat

*Note: Look for quinoa at a health food store or in the grains section of a large supermarket.

For Wave 1, serve with a mixed green salad. For Waves 2 and 3, serve with fresh peach slices.

Wine Pairing: Syrah

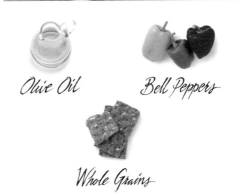

Olive Oil   *Bell Peppers*

Whole Grains

MUSTARD-CRUSTED BEEF TENDERLOIN

*Melt-in-your-mouth beef tenderloin enhanced with the fresh,
sharp flavor of mustard makes this a dish you won't soon forget.*

Prep: 25 minutes **Roast:** 35 minutes **Stand:** 10 minutes **Oven:** 425°F **Makes:** 4 servings

¼ cup coarse-grain mustard

2 teaspoons honey

¾ teaspoon dry mustard

¾ teaspoon freshly ground black pepper

½ teaspoon finely shredded orange peel

½ teaspoon finely shredded lemon peel

1 tablespoon extra-virgin olive oil

1 1-pound beef tenderloin roast

Olive Oil

1. Preheat oven to 425°F. In a small bowl combine coarse-grain mustard, honey, dry mustard, the ¾ teaspoon pepper, the orange peel, and lemon peel; set aside.

2. In a heavy large skillet heat olive oil over medium-high heat. Quickly brown roast on all sides in hot oil (about 2 minutes total). Transfer meat to a rack set in a shallow roasting pan. Spread mustard mixture over top and sides of roast. Insert an oven-going meat thermometer into center of roast.

3. Roast beef for 35 to 45 minutes or until meat thermometer registers 140°F. Cover meat with foil and let stand for 10 to 15 minutes before slicing. The temperature of the meat after standing should be 145°F.

Nutrition facts per serving: 234 cal., 12 g total fat
(3 g sat. fat), 70 mg chol., 533 mg sodium, 3 g carbo.,
0 g fiber, 24 g pro.
Exchanges: 3½ Lean Meat, ½ Fat

*For Wave 1, this is not appropriate. For Waves
2 and 3, serve with roasted beets, a whole grain
roll, and fresh plum wedges.*

Wine Pairing: Merlot

ROASTED PEPPERCORN BEEF WITH FENNEL AND TOMATO SALAD

Roasted beef on top of elegantly seasoned vegetables makes the perfect entrée for entertaining. Red wine vinegar perks up the fennel and tomato salad and contributes flavonoids for antioxidant activity.

Prep: 25 minutes **Cook:** 15 minutes **Roast:** 25 minutes **Stand:** 15 minutes **Oven:** 350°F **Makes:** 4 servings

1 12-ounce beef tenderloin roast or boneless beef top loin roast

Kosher salt

1 tablespoon whole black peppercorns, cracked or crushed

1 tablespoon dried whole green peppercorns, cracked or crushed

2 tablespoons extra-virgin olive oil

6 cloves garlic, minced (1 tablespoon minced)

2 cups thinly sliced fennel

½ cup thin wedges red onion

1 tablespoon chopped fresh thyme

1 teaspoon fennel seeds, crushed

¼ teaspoon kosher salt

⅛ teaspoon freshly ground black pepper

2 cups cherry tomatoes, halved

3 tablespoons red wine vinegar

1 tablespoon chopped fresh flat-leaf parsley

Olive Oil

Tomatoes

1. Preheat oven to 350°F. Trim fat from beef. Season beef with kosher salt. In a small bowl combine black and green peppercorns. Spread peppercorn mixture on a sheet of waxed paper and roll tenderloin roast in peppercorn mixture on all sides to coat.

2. In a large skillet heat 1 tablespoon of the olive oil over medium heat. Add tenderloin roast; cook about 8 minutes or until browned on all sides, turning to brown evenly. Place tenderloin roast on a rack in a shallow roasting pan. Roast, uncovered, for 25 to 30 minutes or until medium-rare doneness (135°F). Cover with foil and let stand for 15 minutes before slicing. The temperature of the meat after standing should be 145°F.

3. Meanwhile, in the same skillet heat the remaining 1 tablespoon olive oil over medium heat. Add garlic; cook about 1 minute or until fragrant. Add fennel, red onion, thyme, fennel seeds, the ¼ teaspoon kosher salt, and the freshly ground black pepper. Cook and stir about 5 minutes or until vegetables are tender. Add the cherry tomatoes, red wine vinegar, and parsley; heat through.

4. Place fennel and tomato salad on a serving platter. Thinly slice the meat; arrange on top of the salad.

Nutrition facts per serving: 239 cal., 13 g total fat (3 g sat. fat), 52 mg chol., 431 mg sodium, 11 g carbo., 3 g fiber, 20 g pro.
Exchanges: 1½ Vegetable, 2½ Lean Meat, 1½ Fat

For Wave 1, serve with cooked bulgur and cucumber slices. For Waves 2 and 3, serve with cooked bulgur and fresh pear slices.

Wine Pairing: Zinfandel

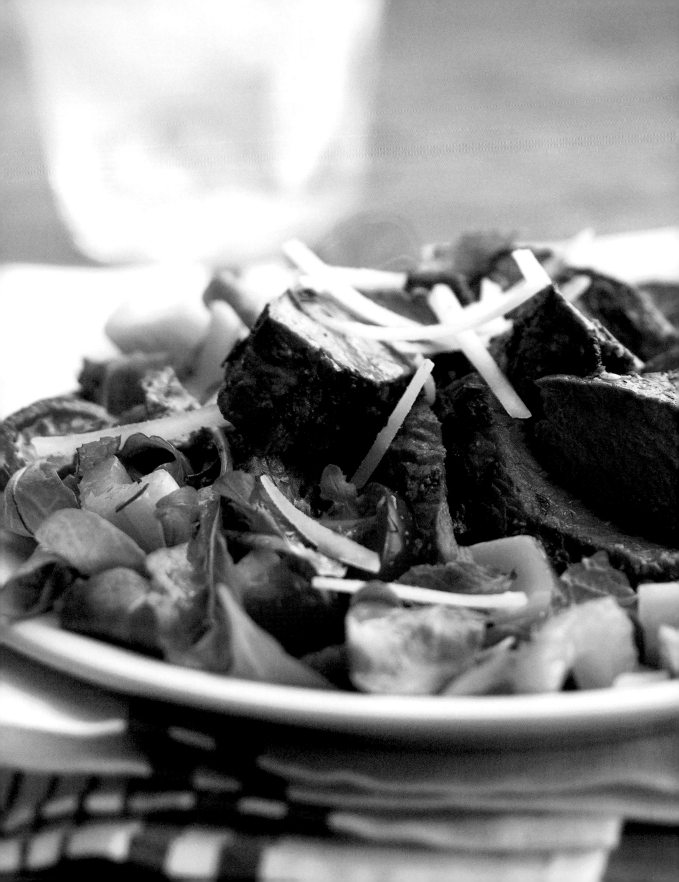

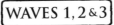

GRILLED WINE COUNTRY BEEF WITH ARUGULA

Although this marinade contains several distinctly flavored ingredients, they fuse harmoniously. Start marinating up to a day in advance to allow the flavors to blend and save you time.

Prep: 15 minutes **Marinate:** 1 to 24 hours **Grill:** 14 minutes **Stand:** 5 minutes **Makes:** 4 servings

4   6-ounce boneless beef sirloin steaks, cut 1 inch thick

Kosher salt

Freshly ground black pepper

¼   cup extra-virgin olive oil

2   tablespoons chopped fresh mint

1   tablespoon chopped fresh rosemary

½   to 1 teaspoon crushed red pepper

2   tablespoons lemon juice

1   tablespoon red wine vinegar

6   cups torn arugula leaves

1   cup thinly sliced celery

1   cup cherry tomatoes, halved

2   tablespoons shredded Parmesan or Asiago cheese

1. Trim fat from steaks. Season steaks with kosher salt and black pepper. Place steaks in a large self-sealing plastic bag set in a shallow dish.

2. For marinade, in a small bowl combine 2 tablespoons of the olive oil, 1 tablespoon of the mint, the rosemary, and crushed red pepper. Pour over steaks. Seal bag; turn to coat steaks. Marinate in the refrigerator for 1 to 24 hours, turning bag occasionally.

3. For dressing, in a screw-top jar combine lemon juice, red wine vinegar, and remaining 2 tablespoons olive oil. Cover and shake well. Season to taste with additional kosher salt and black pepper. Set aside.

4. Drain steaks, discarding marinade. For a charcoal grill, place steaks on the rack of an uncovered grill directly over medium coals. Grill for 14 to 18 minutes for medium-rare doneness (145°F) or 18 to 22 minutes for medium doneness (160°F), turning once halfway through grilling. (For a gas grill, preheat grill. Reduce heat to medium. Place steaks on grill rack over heat. Cover and grill as above.)

5. Remove steaks from grill. Cover with foil and let stand for 5 to 10 minutes. Slice meat across the grain.

6. In a large bowl combine arugula, celery, tomatoes, and the remaining 1 tablespoon mint. Drizzle with the dressing; toss to coat.

7. To serve, divide arugula mixture among four dinner plates; top with meat slices. Sprinkle with Parmesan cheese.

Nutrition facts per serving: 360 cal., 20 g total fat (4 g sat. fat), 105 mg chol., 342 mg sodium, 5 g carbo., 2 g fiber, 39 g pro.
Exchanges: 2 Vegetable, 5 Lean Meat, 1 Fat

For Wave 1, serve with toasted whole grain bread. For Waves 2 and 3, serve with toasted whole grain bread and fresh pear slices.

Wine Pairing: Sangiovese

Olive Oil

Tomatoes

SOUTH AMERICAN FLANK STEAK

Scoring the meat first allows excess fat to drain during cooking and assists with flavor absorption and tenderization while marinating. For less heat in the marinade, just use a couple teaspoons of the adobo sauce and leave out the chipotle peppers.

Prep: 15 minutes **Marinate:** 2 hours **Grill:** 17 minutes **Makes:** 4 servings

1 1-pound beef flank steak

1 cup lightly packed fresh cilantro

⅓ cup orange juice

4 teaspoons red wine vinegar

1 tablespoon extra-virgin olive oil

4 cloves garlic, minced (2 teaspoons minced)

2 teaspoons ground cumin

2 teaspoons ground coriander

1½ to 2 teaspoons finely chopped canned chipotle chile peppers in adobo sauce*

¼ teaspoon kosher salt

¼ teaspoon freshly ground black pepper

Olive Oil

1. Trim fat from steak. Score both sides of steak in a diamond pattern by making shallow cuts at 1-inch intervals. Place steak in a self-sealing plastic bag set in a shallow dish.

2. In a blender combine cilantro, orange juice, vinegar, olive oil, garlic, cumin, coriander, chile peppers, kosher salt, and black pepper. Cover and blend until smooth. Pour orange juice mixture over steak. Seal bag; turn to coat steak. Marinate in the refrigerator for 2 hours, turning bag occasionally.

3. Drain steak, discarding marinade. For a charcoal grill, place steak on the rack of an uncovered grill directly over medium coals. Grill for 17 to 21 minutes or until medium doneness (160°F), turning steak once halfway through grilling. (For a gas grill, preheat grill. Reduce heat to medium. Place steak on grill rack over heat. Cover and grill as above.)

4. To serve, thinly slice steak across the grain.

Nutrition facts per serving: 193 cal., 9 g total fat (3 g sat. fat), 47 mg chol., 126 mg sodium, 2 g carbo., 1 g fiber, 25 g pro.
Exchanges: 3½ Lean Meat

* Note: Because hot chile peppers contain oils that can burn your skin and eyes, wear rubber or plastic gloves when working with them. If your bare hands do touch the chile peppers, wash your hands well with soap and water.

For Wave 1, this is not appropriate. For Waves 2 and 3, serve with cooked quinoa, fresh papaya, and cooked yellow summer squash or zucchini.

Wine Pairing: Zinfandel

CHIPOTLE FLANK STEAK

Tomatillos and chipotle peppers give this dish a Southwestern flair.
Also known as Mexican green tomatoes, tomatillos provide vitamins A and C.

Prep: 35 minutes **Cook:** 10 minutes **Makes:** 6 servings

1½ pounds beef flank steak

½ teaspoon kosher salt

½ teaspoon freshly ground black pepper

2 tablespoons extra-virgin olive oil

1 large onion, thinly sliced

1 large red bell pepper, seeded and cut into thin strips

1 teaspoon ground cumin

1 teaspoon freshly ground black pepper

5 cloves garlic, minced (2½ teaspoons minced)

1¼ cups Roasted Tomatillo-Chipotle Salsa

½ cup chicken broth

Chopped fresh cilantro

1. Trim fat from steak. Score both sides of steak in a diamond pattern by making shallow diagonal cuts at 1-inch intervals. Cut steak into 4 equal pieces. Season steak pieces with kosher salt and the ½ teaspoon black pepper.

2. In a 10-inch skillet heat 1 tablespoon olive oil over medium-high heat. Add steak pieces. Cook about 5 minutes or until well browned, turning to brown evenly. Remove steak pieces from skillet; set aside.

3. Add the remaining 1 tablespoon olive oil, the onion, and bell pepper to skillet. Cook and stir about 3 minutes or until crisp-tender and lightly browned. Add the cumin, the 1 teaspoon black pepper, and the garlic. Cook and stir for 1 minute. Add Roasted Tomatillo-Chipotle Salsa. Bring to boiling; reduce heat. Simmer, uncovered, for 5 minutes, stirring occasionally. Add chicken broth; return to boiling. Add steak pieces to skillet. Reduce heat. Cover and simmer for 10 to 15 minutes or until desired doneness

(145°F for medium-rare doneness or 160°F for medium doneness).

4. Transfer steak pieces to a cutting board; thinly slice against the grain. Transfer to serving plates or shallow bowls. Spoon salsa mixture over and around the meat. Sprinkle individual servings with cilantro.

Nutrition facts per serving: 243 cal., 12 g total fat (3 g sat. fat), 47 mg chol., 378 mg sodium, 8 g carbo., 1 g fiber, 26 g pro.
Exchanges: 1 Vegetable, 3½ Very Lean Meat, ½ Fat

Roasted Tomatillo-Chipotle Salsa: Preheat oven to 450°F. Remove husks from 1½ pounds fresh tomatillos; rinse well. Arrange the tomatillos and 4 unpeeled garlic cloves in a shallow baking pan. Bake, uncovered, about 20 minutes or until tomatillos and garlic are softened and charred, stirring once. Cool. When cool enough to handle, squeeze garlic paste from cloves. In a food processor or blender combine the tomatillos and any juices, the garlic paste, and 1 canned chipotle chile pepper in adobo sauce.° Cover and process or blend until smooth. Add ½ of a medium onion, cut into wedges; 2 tablespoons packed fresh cilantro; 1 tablespoon lime juice; and ½ teaspoon kosher salt. Cover and process or blend just until onion is chopped. Use immediately or cover and chill for up to 2 weeks. Serve leftover salsa with cooked beef or pork. Makes about 3 cups.

*See note, page 76

For Wave 1, serve with cooked brown rice and steamed cauliflower. For Waves 2 and 3, serve with cooked brown rice and fresh grapefruit.

Wine Pairing: Pinot Noir

Olive Oil

Bell Peppers

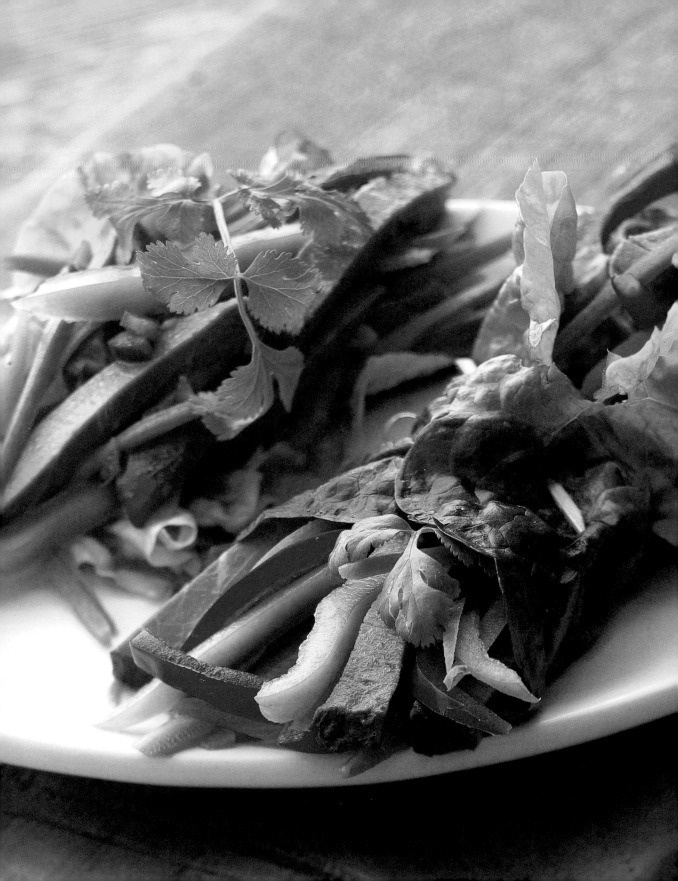

THAI ROAST BEEF LETTUCE ROLLS

*When you're looking for an enticing meal but don't have a lot of time, enjoy these
Thai-inspired wraps. Holding true to Thai tradition, they call for fish sauce,
an essential Thai ingredient that adds a salty, piquant flavor.*

Start to Finish: 30 minutes **Makes:** 4 servings

2	tablespoons lime juice
1	tablespoon bottled fish sauce
1	tablespoon water
1½	teaspoons honey
2	cloves garlic, minced (1 teaspoon minced)
1	teaspoon finely chopped fresh jalapeño or serrano chile pepper*
1	pound cooked roast beef, cut into thin strips
8	leaves red leaf lettuce
1½	cups red and/or green bell pepper strips
1½	cups bite-size carrot strips
16	sprigs fresh cilantro and/or mint

1. In a medium bowl whisk together lime juice, fish sauce, the water, honey, garlic, and chile pepper. Add beef strips; toss well.

2. Arrange 2 lettuce leaves on each of four dinner plates. Top lettuce with meat strips, pepper strips, carrot strips, and cilantro and/or mint. Drizzle with any remaining lime mixture. Roll up lettuce leaves. Serve immediately.

Nutrition facts per serving: 281 cal., 15 g total fat (5 g sat. fat), 80 mg chol., 634 mg sodium, 10 g carbo., 2 g fiber, 28 g pro.
Exchanges: 2 Vegetable, 3½ Lean Meat, 1 Fat

*See note, page 76

For Wave 1, this is not appropriate. For Waves 2 and 3, serve with cooked soba noodles and fresh apple slices.

Wine Pairing: rosé

Bell Peppers

TERIYAKI BEEF SPIRALS

Chopped water chestnuts, a common ingredient in Asian cooking, give the fresh spinach filling an added crunch. The toothpicks and skewers help hold the spirals together as they broil.

Prep: 30 minutes **Broil:** 12 minutes **Makes:** 5 servings

1 cup lightly packed fresh spinach leaves

½ cup finely chopped water chestnuts

¼ cup thinly sliced green onions

2 teaspoons minced fresh ginger

4 cloves garlic, minced (2 teaspoons minced)

¼ cup bottled reduced-sodium teriyaki sauce

1 1¼-pound beef flank steak

Kosher salt

Freshly ground black pepper

Spinach

1. Remove stems from spinach leaves. Layer leaves on top of each other; slice crosswise into thin strips. In a medium bowl combine spinach, water chestnuts, green onions, ginger, garlic, and 2 tablespoons of the teriyaki sauce.

2. Trim fat from steak. Score both sides of steak in a diamond pattern by making shallow diagonal cuts at 1-inch intervals. Place steak between 2 sheets of plastic wrap. Working from center to edges, use the flat side of a meat mallet to pound the steak into a 12×8-inch rectangle. Remove plastic wrap. Season steak lightly with kosher salt and pepper.

3. Spread spinach mixture over steak. Starting from a long side, roll rectangle into a spiral. Starting ½ inch from one end, secure with wooden toothpicks at 1-inch intervals. Cut between toothpicks into 10 pinwheels. Thread two pinwheels onto each of five long metal skewers. Brush with some of the remaining 2 tablespoons teriyaki sauce.

4. Place skewers on the rack of an unheated broiler pan. Broil 3 to 4 inches from heat for 12 to 14 minutes or until medium doneness, turning once and brushing with teriyaki sauce halfway through broiling time. Discard any remaining teriyaki sauce. Remove toothpicks and skewers.

Nutrition facts per serving: 207 cal., 8 g total fat (4 g sat. fat), 46 mg chol., 525 mg sodium, 5 g carbo., 1 g fiber, 26 g pro.
Exchanges: ½ Vegetable, 3½ Lean Meat

For Wave 1, serve with a spinach salad and cooked soba noodles. For Waves 2 and 3, serve with a spinach salad, cooked soba noodles, and fresh apricot slices.

Wine Pairing: Zinfandel

GARDEN POT ROAST

The long baking time for this traditional comfort food gives the flavors time to mingle, resulting in moist, succulent meat. Be sure the vegetables you choose are Wave appropriate.

Prep: 25 minutes **Bake:** 1½ hours + 1 hour **Oven:** 325°F **Makes:** 8 servings

1 3-pound boneless beef bottom round rump roast

Kosher salt

Freshly ground black pepper

1 tablespoon extra-virgin olive oil

1 cup dry red wine

1 14-ounce can beef broth

½ cup coarsely chopped onion

½ teaspoon dried marjoram, crushed

½ teaspoon dried thyme, crushed

2 cloves garlic, minced (1 teaspoon minced)

6 cups fresh vegetables cut into 1- to 1½-inch pieces (such as winter squash, carrots, parsnips, and/or green beans)

2 tablespoons cold water

1 tablespoon cornstarch

Olive Oil

1. Preheat oven to 325°F. Trim fat from roast. Season roast with kosher salt and pepper. In a 6-quart oven-going Dutch oven brown roast in hot olive oil for 5 minutes, turning to brown evenly. Remove roast from Dutch oven; set aside. Carefully drain fat from Dutch oven. Add wine to Dutch oven; bring to boiling. Boil gently, uncovered, for 8 to 10 minutes or until wine is reduced to ½ cup. Return roast to Dutch oven. Pour broth over roast. Add onion, marjoram, thyme, and garlic. Bake, covered, for 1½ hours.

2. Add desired fresh vegetables. Cover and bake about 1 hour more or until meat and vegetables are tender. Transfer meat and vegetables to a serving platter; reserve cooking juices in the Dutch oven. Cover meat and vegetables with foil to keep warm.

3. For gravy, strain cooking juices into a 4-cup glass measure. Skim fat from cooking juices; return 1¼ cups of the cooking juices to Dutch oven (discard remaining juices). In a small bowl stir together the cold water and cornstarch. Stir into cooking juices in Dutch oven. Cook and stir until thickened and bubbly. Cook and stir for 2 minutes more. Season to taste with kosher salt and pepper.

4. Slice meat. Spoon some of the gravy over meat and vegetables. Pass remaining gravy.

Nutrition facts per serving: 316 cal., 9 g total fat (2 g sat. fat), 98 mg chol., 433 mg sodium, 12 g carbo., 3 g fiber, 39 g pro.
Exchanges: ½ Vegetable, ½ Starch, 5 Very Lean Meat, 2 Fat

For Wave 1, this is not appropriate. For Waves 2 and 3, serve with a whole grain roll and fresh berries.

Wine Pairing: Merlot

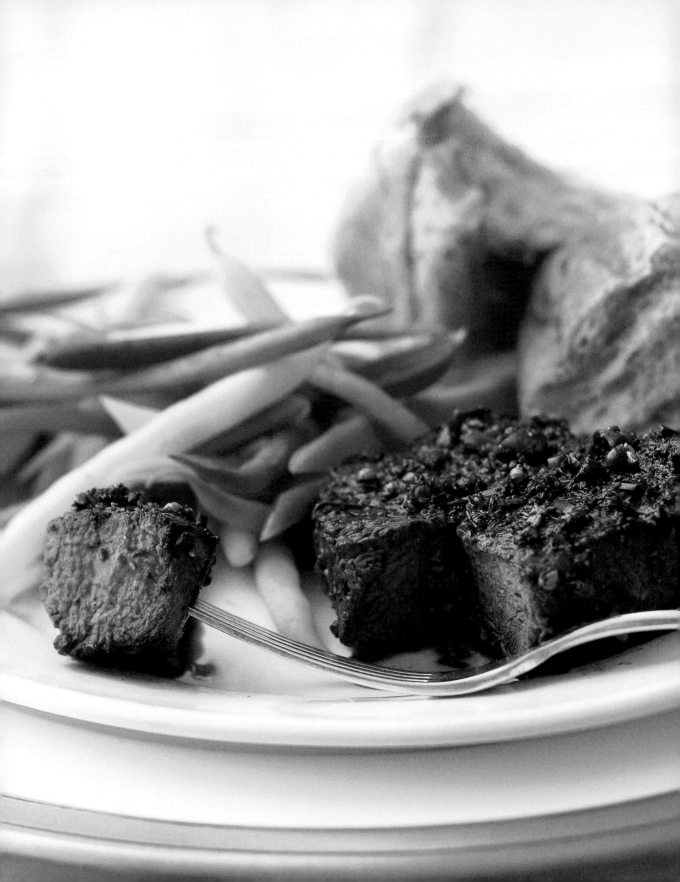

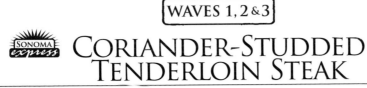

CORIANDER-STUDDED TENDERLOIN STEAK

Crushed coriander seeds bestow a slightly sweet citrus flavor upon these tender steaks, making them irresistible.

Prep: 10 minutes **Broil:** 12 minutes **Makes:** 4 servings

4 3- to 4-ounce beef tenderloin steaks, cut 1 inch thick

Kosher salt

1 tablespoon reduced-sodium soy sauce

1 tablespoon extra-virgin olive oil

1 tablespoon chopped fresh chives

2 cloves garlic, minced (1 teaspoon minced)

½ teaspoon coriander seeds or cumin seeds, crushed

½ teaspoon celery seeds

½ teaspoon coarsely ground black pepper

Olive Oil

1. Preheat broiler. Trim fat from steaks. Season steaks with kosher salt. In a small bowl combine soy sauce, olive oil, chives, garlic, coriander seeds or cumin seeds, celery seeds, and pepper. Brush mixture onto both sides of each steak.

2. Place steaks on the unheated rack of a broiler pan. Broil 3 to 4 inches from heat for 12 to 14 minutes for medium-rare doneness (145°F) or 15 to 18 minutes for medium doneness (160°F) turning once halfway through broiling time.

Nutrition facts per serving: 164 cal., 9 g total fat (3 g sat. fat), 42 mg chol., 256 mg sodium, 1 g carbo., 0 g fiber, 18 g pro.
Exchanges: 2½ Lean Meat, ½ Fat

For Wave 1, serve with cooked green or wax beans and a whole grain roll. For Waves 2 and 3, serve with cooked green or wax beans, a whole grain roll, and fresh grapes.

Wine Pairing: Merlot

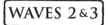
ROUND STEAK WITH VEGETABLES

For a busy cook, nothing beats the convenience of a slow cooker. The slow cooking method is ideal for round steak because it goes in as a tougher cut of meat and comes out moist and succulent.

Prep: 15 minutes **Cook:** Low 8 hours, High 4 hours **Makes:** 4 servings

1½ pounds boneless beef round steak, cut ¾ to 1 inch thick

Kosher salt

Freshly ground black pepper

2 cups packaged peeled baby carrots

1 large onion, cut into wedges

1 4½-ounce jar (drained weight) sliced mushrooms, drained

1 14½-ounce can diced tomatoes with basil, oregano, and garlic, undrained

3 tablespoons Italian-style tomato paste

1 tablespoon Worcestershire sauce

1 small zucchini, halved lengthwise and sliced (1 cup)

Tomatoes

1. Trim fat from meat. Cut steak into four serving-size pieces; season steaks with kosher salt and pepper. Place meat in a 3½- or 4-quart slow cooker. Top meat with carrots, onion, and mushrooms.

2. In a medium bowl stir together undrained tomatoes, tomato paste, and Worcestershire sauce. Pour tomato mixture over meat and vegetables.

3. Cover and cook on low-heat setting for 8 to 9 hours or on high-heat setting for 4 to 4½ hours, adding zucchini for the last 30 minutes of cooking.

Nutrition facts per serving: 336 cal., 8 g total fat (2 g sat. fat), 98 mg chol., 1,008 mg sodium, 24 g carbo., 5 g fiber, 41 g pro.
Exchanges: 4 Vegetable, 4½ Very Lean Meat, 1½ Fat

For Wave 1, this is not appropriate. For Waves 2 and 3, serve with cooked multigrain pasta and fresh grapes.

Wine Pairing: Cabernet

STEAK WITH HERB-PEPPER MUSTARD

A bit of French flavor from Dijon mustard and thyme adds instant excitement to this popular cut of beef

Prep: 30 minutes **Grill:** 21 minutes **Stand:** 20 minutes **Makes:** 4 servings

2 medium red bell peppers, quartered lengthwise

Extra-virgin olive oil

2 tablespoons chopped fresh thyme or 2 teaspoons dried thyme, crushed

1 tablespoon Dijon-style mustard

3 cloves garlic, minced (1½ teaspoons minced)

2 T-bone steaks, cut 1 inch thick (about 2¼ pounds total)

¼ teaspoon kosher salt

¼ teaspoon freshly ground black pepper

Olive Oil

Bell Peppers

1. Brush bell peppers with olive oil. For a charcoal grill, place peppers, cut sides up, on the rack of an uncovered grill directly over medium-hot coals. Grill about 10 minutes or until pepper skins are blistered and dark. (For a gas grill, preheat grill. Reduce heat to medium-hot. Place peppers, cut sides up, on grill rack over heat. Cover and grill as above.)

2. Wrap peppers in foil and let stand for 20 minutes. Remove and discard pepper skins. Cut 2 pepper pieces lengthwise into thin strips; set aside. In a blender or food processor combine the remaining pepper pieces, 1 tablespoon of the fresh thyme or 1 teaspoon of the dried thyme, the Dijon mustard, and 1 clove of the garlic. Cover and blend or process until smooth.

3. Meanwhile, trim fat from steaks. For rub, in a small bowl combine the remaining 1 tablespoon fresh thyme or 1 teaspoon dried thyme, the remaining 2 cloves garlic, the kosher salt, and black pepper. Sprinkle mixture evenly over steaks; rub in with your fingers. Add steaks to grill. Grill for 11 to 14 minutes for medium-rare doneness (145°F) or 13 to 16 minutes for medium doneness (160°F), turning once halfway through grilling.

4. Top the steaks with the grilled pepper strips. Serve with the mustard mixture.

Nutrition facts per serving: 250 cal., 11 g total fat (3 g sat. fat), 68 mg chol., 295 mg sodium, 5 g carbo., 1 g fiber, 31 g pro.
Exchanges: ½ Vegetable, 4½ Lean Meat

For Wave 1, serve with a whole grain roll and steamed cauliflower. For Waves 2 and 3, serve with a whole grain roll and fresh cantaloupe.

Wine Pairing: Cabernet Sauvignon

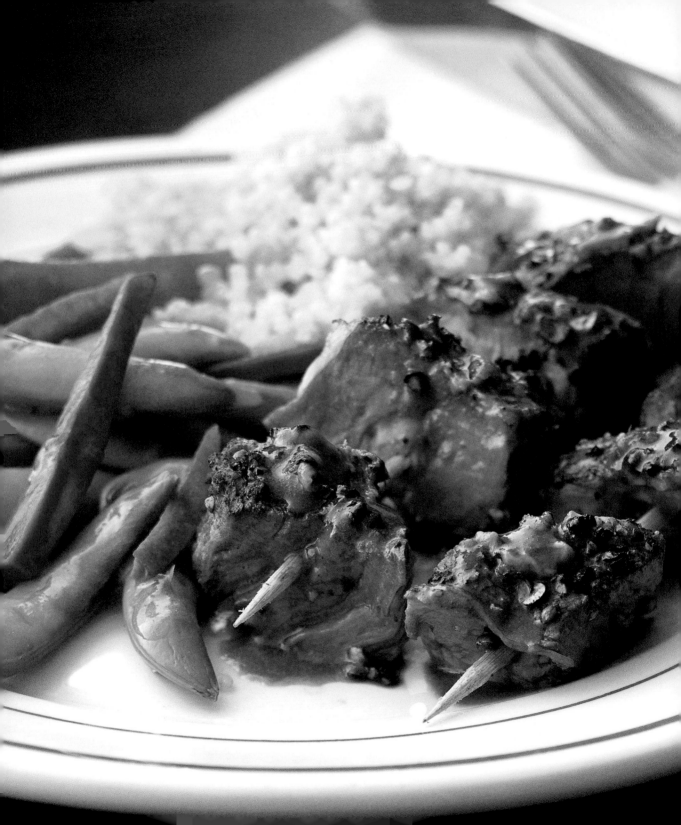

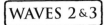
PEPPERCORN STEAK KABOBS

The inventive combination of molasses and peppercorns gives this beautifully colored dish bold flavor. Using a mild-flavored molasses will ensure its flavor doesn't overpower the dish.

Start to Finish: 35 minutes **Makes:** 4 servings

4 8- to 10-inch wooden skewers

2 6-ounce boneless beef ribeye steaks or top sirloin steaks, cut about 1 inch thick

1 tablespoon multicolor peppercorns, crushed

½ teaspoon kosher salt

3 tablespoons extra-virgin olive oil

1 tablespoon mild-flavored molasses

¼ teaspoon finely shredded lemon peel

1½ teaspoons lemon juice

2 cups fresh sugar snap peas

½ cup bite-size carrot strips

Lemon peel strips (optional)

Olive Oil

1. Soak skewers in enough water to cover for at least 1 hour before using. Preheat broiler. Trim fat from steaks. Using your fingers, press the crushed peppercorns and kosher salt onto both sides of each steak. Cut steaks into 1-inch cubes. Thread steak cubes onto skewers, leaving a ¼-inch space between each piece.

2. Place skewers on the unheated rack of a broiler pan. Broil 4 to 5 inches from the heat for 10 to 12 minutes or until desired doneness (145°F for medium-rare doneness or 160°F for medium doneness), turning once halfway through broiling time.

3. Meanwhile, in a small bowl combine oil, molasses, finely shredded lemon peel, and lemon juice. Set aside.

4. Remove strings and tips from sugar snap peas. In a covered medium saucepan cook sugar snap peas and carrot in a small amount of salted, boiling water for 2 to 4 minutes or until crisp-tender. Drain well. Stir in 1 tablespoon of the molasses mixture.

5. To serve, drizzle remaining molasses mixture evenly over steaks and serve with vegetable mixture. If desired, garnish with lemon peel strips.

Nutrition facts per serving: 260 cal., 17 g total fat (4 g sat. fat), 50 mg chol., 301 mg sodium, 9 g carbo., 2 g fiber, 18 g pro.
Exchanges: 1 Vegetable, 2½ Lean Meat, 2 Fat

For Wave 1, this is not appropriate. For Waves 2 and 3, serve with cooked quinoa and fresh orange slices.

Wine Pairing: Sauvignon Blanc

SALSA STEAK

This salsa-smothered steak calls for lots of fresh, brightly colored vegetables.
For more Mediterranean flavor, try Italian seasoning in place of the chili powder.

Prep: 20 minutes **Bake:** 45 minutes **Oven:** 350°F **Makes:** 4 to 6 servings

1   to 1½ pounds boneless beef round steak, cut ½ inch thick

Kosher salt

Freshly ground black pepper

1   tablespoon canola oil

1½ cups sliced fresh mushrooms

1   medium green bell pepper, cut into bite-size strips

1   medium onion, sliced

1   8-ounce can tomato sauce

1   2¼-ounce can sliced pitted ripe olives, drained (optional)

2   to 3 teaspoons chili powder*

Tomatoes

Bell Peppers

1. Preheat oven to 350°F. Trim fat from meat. Season both sides of meat with kosher salt and black pepper. Cut meat into 4 to 6 serving-size pieces. In a large skillet brown meat in hot oil, turning once. Transfer meat to a 2-quart square baking dish.

2. In the same skillet cook and stir mushrooms, bell pepper, and onion over medium heat for 5 to 8 minutes or until tender (add more oil if necessary). Stir in tomato sauce, olives (if desired), and chili powder. Cook and stir until bubbly.

3. Pour mushroom mixture over meat in baking dish. Cover and bake about 45 minutes or until meat is tender.

Nutrition facts per serving: 223 cal., 9 g total fat (2 g sat. fat), 54 mg chol., 454 mg sodium, 8 g carbo., 2 g fiber, 27 g pro.
Exchanges: 1½ Vegetable, 3½ Very Lean Meat, 1½ Fat

*Note: Another time opt for an Italian-flavored dish by substituting 1 to 1½ teaspoons dried Italian seasoning, crushed, for the chili powder.

For Wave 1, serve with cooked brown rice and steamed fresh broccoli. For Waves 2 and 3, serve with cooked brown rice and fresh peach slices.

Wine Pairing: sparkling semisweet

PINEAPPLE-TERIYAKI BEEF

Nothing goes to waste in this dish; even the leftover marinade becomes a delectable steak sauce. The marinade perfectly pairs teriyaki and pineapple to intensify flavor and can be prepared a day in advance so your steak can soak overnight.

Prep: 15 minutes **Broil:** 18 minutes **Marinate:** 6 to 24 hours **Makes:** 6 to 8 servings

1   2-pound boneless beef top round steak, cut 1½ inches thick

1   8-ounce can crushed pineapple (juice pack)

2   tablespoons finely chopped green onion

2   tablespoons reduced-sodium teriyaki sauce

2   cloves garlic, minced (1 teaspoon minced)

1   teaspoon grated fresh ginger

1   teaspoon toasted sesame oil

¼   cup sliced green onions

1   tablespoon sesame seeds, toasted

1. Trim fat from steak. Place steak in a self-sealing plastic bag set in a shallow dish. Drain pineapple, reserving juice. Cover and refrigerate pineapple for sauce.

2. For marinade, in a small bowl stir together the reserved pineapple juice, the 2 tablespoons green onion, teriyaki sauce, garlic, ginger, and sesame oil.

3. Pour marinade over steak. Seal bag; turn to coat steak. Marinate in the refrigerator for 6 to 24 hours, turning bag occasionally.

4. Drain steak, reserving the marinade. Place steak on the unheated rack of a broiler pan. Broil 4 to 5 inches from heat for 18 to 20 minutes total for medium-rare doneness (145°F), turning once halfway through broiling.

5. Meanwhile, for sauce, in a small saucepan combine the reserved marinade and the pineapple. Bring to boiling; reduce heat. Simmer, uncovered, for 5 minutes. Remove from heat. Serve sauce with steak. Sprinkle with ¼ cup green onions and sesame seeds to serve.

Nutrition facts per serving: 281 cal., 10 g total fat (3 g sat. fat), 66 mg chol., 235 mg sodium, 8 g carbo., 1 g fiber, 38 g pro.
Exchanges: ½ Fruit, 5 Very Lean Meat, 1½ Fat

For Wave 1, this is not appropriate. For Waves 2 and 3, serve with cooked soba noodles, steamed carrots, and fresh kiwifruit.

Wine Pairing: Sauvignon Blanc

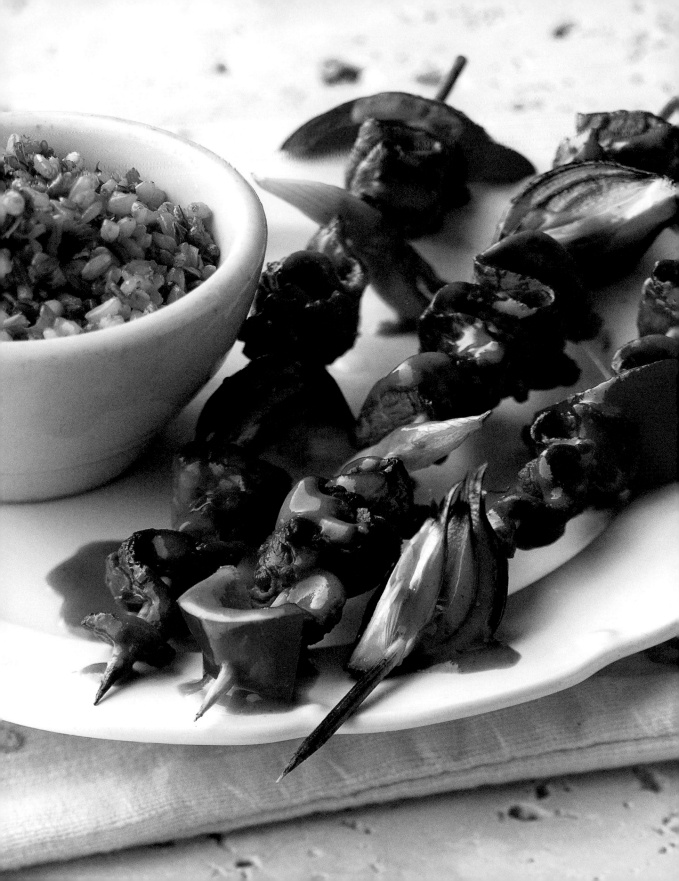

BEEF SATAY WITH PEANUT SAUCE

Staying true to its Indonesian roots, this savory beef satay is skewered and served with a warm peanut sauce, perfect for dipping. For simplified preparation, partially freeze your steak to make slicing easier.

Prep: 25 minutes **Marinate:** 30 minutes **Broil:** 4 minutes **Makes:** 5 servings

1 1- to 1¼-pound beef flank steak

⅓ cup light teriyaki sauce

½ teaspoon bottled hot pepper sauce

½ of a medium red onion, cut into thin wedges

4 green onions, cut into 1-inch pieces

1 red or green bell pepper, cut into ¾-inch chunks

3 tablespoons peanut butter

3 tablespoons water

2 tablespoons light teriyaki sauce

Bell Peppers

1. If desired, partially freeze steak for easier slicing. For satay, trim fat from steak. Cut steak crosswise into thin slices. For marinade, in a medium bowl combine the ⅓ cup teriyaki sauce and ¼ teaspoon of the hot pepper sauce. Add steak; toss to coat. Cover and marinate in the refrigerator for 30 minutes. If using wooden skewers, cook them in water for 30 minutes before using.

2. Drain steak, reserving marinade. On wooden or metal skewers, alternately thread steak strips (accordion style), onion wedges, green onion pieces, and bell pepper. Brush with reserved marinade. Discard any remaining marinade.

3. Place skewers on the unheated rack of a broiler pan. Broil 4 to 5 inches from the heat about 4 minutes or until meat is slightly pink in center, turning once.

4. For peanut sauce, in a small saucepan combine peanut butter, the water, the 2 tablespoons teriyaki sauce, and the remaining ¼ teaspoon hot pepper sauce. Cook and stir over medium heat just until smooth and heated through.

5. Serve satay with warm peanut sauce.

Nutrition facts per serving: 230 cal., 10 g total fat (3 g sat. fat), 38 mg chol., 730 mg sodium, 10 g carbo., 2 g fiber, 24 g pro.
Exchanges: ½ Vegetable, ½ Other Carbo., 3 Lean Meat, ½ Fat

For Wave 1, serve with cooked brown rice and a spinach salad. For Waves 2 and 3, serve with cooked brown rice, a spinach salad, and fresh pineapple.

Wine Pairing: sparkling white or sparkling red

CHARD-TOPPED STEAKS

A simple topping of Swiss chard pumps up the flavor, color, and aroma of these delectable, meaty tenderloins. Chard also contains oodles of health-promoting nutrients such as vitamins A, C, K, and E, iron, potassium, magnesium, and copper.

Prep: 20 minutes **Broil:** 12 minutes **Makes:** 4 servings

1 slice bacon, chopped

4 4-ounce beef tenderloin steaks, cut 1 inch thick

Kosher salt

Freshly ground black pepper

3 cups very thinly sliced Swiss chard leaves (4 ounces)

4 cloves garlic, minced (2 teaspoons minced)

1 cup seeded, chopped tomato

2 teaspoons chopped fresh thyme

⅛ teaspoon kosher salt

⅛ teaspoon freshly ground black pepper

Tomatoes

1. In a large skillet cook bacon over medium heat until crisp. Remove from skillet, reserving drippings. Crumble bacon; set aside. Remove skillet from heat; set aside.

2. Preheat broiler. Season steaks with kosher salt and pepper. Place steaks on the unheated rack of a broiler pan. Broil 4 to 5 inches from the heat for 12 to 14 minutes for medium-rare doneness (145°F) or 15 to 18 minutes for medium doneness (160°F), turning once halfway through broiling time.

3. Meanwhile, in the large skillet cook and stir Swiss chard and garlic in reserved drippings over medium heat for 4 to 6 minutes or just until tender. Stir in tomato, crumbled bacon, thyme, the ⅛ teaspoon kosher salt, and the ⅛ teaspoon pepper. To serve, spoon Swiss chard mixture on top of steaks.

Nutrition facts per serving: 238 cal., 13 g total fat (4 g sat. fat), 76 mg chol., 372 mg sodium, 4 g carbo., 1 g fiber, 26 g pro.
Exchanges: 1 Vegetable, 3½ Lean Meat, ½ Fat

For Wave 1, serve with a tossed green salad and cooked barley. For Waves 2 and 3, serve with a tossed green salad, cooked barley, and fresh berries.

Wine Pairing: Pinot Noir

ROASTED GARLIC STEAK

The technique of roasting the garlic, basil, and rosemary melds their distinct flavors to give the steak an incredible depth of flavor.

Prep: 15 minutes **Grill:** 30 minutes **Makes:** 6 servings

1   or 2 whole garlic bulb(s)

3   to 4 teaspoons chopped fresh basil or
    1 teaspoon dried basil, crushed

1   tablespoon chopped fresh rosemary or
    1 teaspoon dried rosemary, crushed

2   tablespoons extra-virgin olive oil

1½ pounds boneless beef ribeye steaks or top
    sirloin steak, cut 1 inch thick

1   to 2 teaspoons cracked black pepper

½   teaspoon kosher salt

1. Using a sharp knife, cut off the top ½ inch from each garlic bulb to expose the ends of the individual cloves. Leaving garlic bulb(s) whole, remove any loose, papery outer layers.

2. Fold a 20×18-inch piece of heavy foil in half crosswise. Trim into a 10-inch square. Place garlic bulb(s), cut side(s) up, in center of foil square. Sprinkle garlic with basil and rosemary; drizzle with oil. Bring up 2 opposite edges of foil and seal with a double fold. Fold remaining edges together to enclose garlic, leaving space for steam to build.

3. For a charcoal grill, place garlic packet on the rack of an uncovered grill directly over medium coals. Grill about 30 minutes or until garlic feels soft when packet is squeezed, turning garlic occasionally.

4. Meanwhile, trim fat from steaks. Season both sides of steaks with pepper and kosher salt; rub in with your fingers. While garlic is grilling, add steaks to grill. For ribeye steaks, grill 11 to 15 minutes for medium-rare doneness (145°F) or 14 to 18 minutes for medium doneness (160°F), turning once halfway through grilling. For sirloin steak, grill 14 to 18 minutes for medium-rare

doneness (145°F) or 18 to 22 minutes for medium doneness (160°F), turning once halfway through grilling. (For a gas grill, preheat grill. Reduce heat to medium. Place garlic, then steaks on grill rack over heat. Cover and grill as above.)

5. To serve, cut steaks into 6 serving-size pieces. Remove garlic from foil, reserving the oil mixture. Squeeze garlic pulp from garlic cloves onto steaks. Mash pulp slightly with a fork; spread over steaks. Drizzle with the reserved oil mixture.

Nutrition facts per serving: 227 cal., 13 g total fat (4 g sat. fat), 66 mg chol., 223 mg sodium, 2 g carbo., 0 g fiber, 23 g pro.
Exchanges: 3½ Lean Meat, 1 Fat

For Wave 1, serve with a spinach salad and cooked multigrain pasta. For Waves 2 and 3, serve with Golden Vegetable Gratin (page 253), cooked multigrain pasta, and fresh pear slices.

Wine Pairing: Pinot Noir

Olive Oil

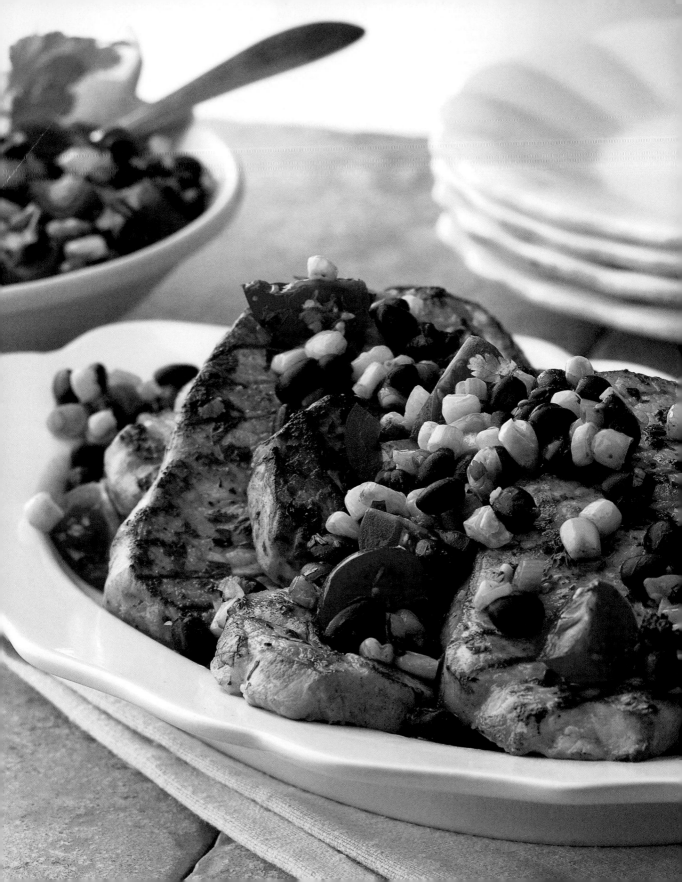

Pork Dinners

Pork is an eager flavor absorber, so it's easy to make even
the leanest cuts of pork burst with taste. See for yourself
when you try the many spice rubs and relishes used
in these recipes. Pork also pairs well with other taste-
enhancing companions common to the Sonoma region—
such as figs, olives, cranberries, toasted almonds, and port.

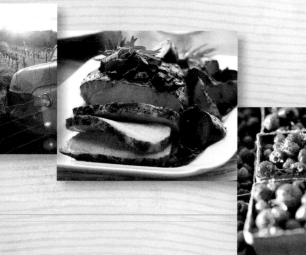
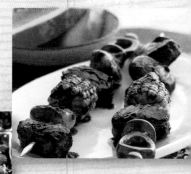

GREEK-STUFFED ROASTED PORK LOIN

*Fresh mint, parsley, roasted red peppers, and feta cheese add a lot of flavor to this simple dish.
Serve it with kale for a bounty of beneficial nutrients such as
vitamins A and C, iron, folic acid, and calcium.*

Prep: 25 minutes **Roast:** 1 hour **Stand:** 10 minutes **Oven:** 325°F **Makes:** 8 servings

1 2- to 2½-pound boneless pork top loin
   roast (single loin)

1 tablespoon chopped fresh mint or dill

1 tablespoon chopped fresh flat-leaf parsley

   Kosher salt

   Freshly ground black pepper

1 12-ounce jar roasted red bell
   peppers, drained

½ cup crumbled feta cheese (2 ounces)

2 cloves garlic, minced (1 teaspoon minced)

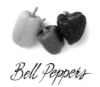

Bell Peppers

1. Preheat oven to 325°F. To butterfly the pork roast, make a lengthwise cut down the center of the roast, cutting to within ½ inch of the opposite side, to form a "V." Spread roast open. Make a parallel slit on each side of the original cut. Open meat to lie flat. Place between 2 pieces of plastic wrap. Working from center to edges, pound with the flat side of a meat mallet to ½-inch thickness. Remove plastic wrap.

2. Sprinkle mint and parsley on pounded side of pork loin. Season pork with kosher salt and pepper. If necessary, split roasted bell peppers to lie flat. Arrange peppers in an even layer on top of the meat. In a small bowl combine feta cheese and garlic. Sprinkle over bell peppers on pork loin. Roll up, starting from a short side; tie with 100%-cotton string at 1½-inch intervals. Season with kosher salt and black pepper.

3. Place roast on a rack in a shallow roasting pan. Insert an oven-going meat thermometer into center of roast. Roast for 1 to 1½ hours or until the thermometer registers 155°F. Cover with foil and let stand for 10 minutes before slicing. The temperature of the meat after standing should be 160°F.

Nutrition facts per serving: 196 cal., 8 g total fat
(3 g sat. fat), 68 mg chol., 181 mg sodium, 2 g carbo.,
1 g fiber, 26 g pro.
Exchanges: ½ Vegetable, 3½ Very Lean Meat, 1½ Fat

*For Wave 1, serve with Roasted Ratatouille
(page 204), steamed kale, and cooked multigrain
pasta. For Waves 2 and 3, serve with Roasted
Ratatouille (page 204), cooked multigrain pasta,
and fresh berries.*

Wine Pairing: Pinot Blanc

PORK WITH APPLES IN CIDER SAUCE

The speckled green skin of Granny Smith apples and their crisp, tart flesh hold up under heat, making them ideal for cooking. Their warm scent is sure to lure anyone around into the kitchen.

Prep: 25 minutes **Bake:** 20 minutes **Cook:** 10 minutes **Oven:** 350°F **Makes:** 4 servings

4   boneless pork loin chops, cut ¾ inch thick (1¼ to 1½ pounds total)

Kosher salt

Freshly ground black pepper

2   tablespoons extra-virgin olive oil

3   medium Granny Smith apples, peeled, cored, and cut into ½-inch-thick slices

1   cup reduced-sodium chicken broth

1   cinnamon stick

1   teaspoon cornstarch

1   teaspoon cold water

Olive Oil

1. Preheat oven to 350°F. Trim fat from meat. Season chops with kosher salt and pepper.

2. In a large skillet cook chops in hot oil for 4 to 6 minutes or until browned, turning to brown evenly. Remove chops from skillet. Set aside.

3. Add apples to the hot skillet; cook and stir about 5 minutes or just until apple slices are browned and tender. Carefully add chicken broth and cinnamon stick to the skillet. Cook and stir for 2 minutes more. Using a slotted spoon, transfer apple slices to a 2-quart rectangular baking dish. Place browned chops atop apples in dish. Pour broth (with stick cinnamon) over pork chops.

4. Cover and bake about 20 minutes or until pork is done (160°F) and juices run clear. Remove the chops from the baking dish; cover and keep warm.

5. Discard cinnamon stick. Spoon the apple mixture into a medium saucepan. Stir together the cornstarch and the cold water; stir into mixture in saucepan. Cook and stir over medium heat until slightly thickened and bubbly; cook and stir for 2 minutes more. Serve chops with apple mixture.

Nutrition facts per serving: 308 cal., 14 g total fat (3 g sat. fat), 89 mg chol., 357 mg sodium, 13 g carbo., 1 g fiber, 32 g pro.
Exchanges: 1 Fruit, 4½ Very Lean Meat, 2 Fat

For Wave 1, this is not appropriate. For Waves 2 and 3, serve with cooked wild rice and steamed green beans.

Wine Pairing: Pinot Noir

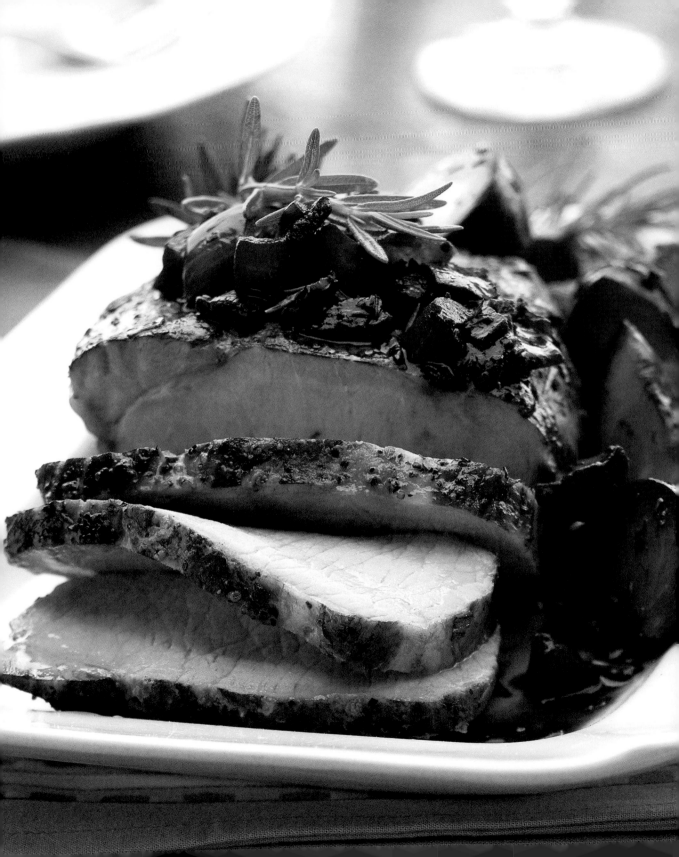

Sonoma Plum and Rosemary Pork Roast

With the many varieties of plums available, you can experiment with the flavor of this recipe every time you make it. No matter which plum variety you choose, its flavor will enhance the pork roast.

Prep: 35 minutes **Bake:** 20 minutes + 20 minutes **Stand:** 15 minutes **Oven:** 300°F **Makes:** 6 servings

1　2-pound boneless pork top loin roast (single loin)

　　Kosher salt

　　Freshly ground black pepper

1　tablespoon extra-virgin olive oil

1　medium onion, chopped

1　medium carrot, chopped

2　tablespoons chopped fresh rosemary

2　cloves garlic, minced (1 teaspoon minced)

1½　cups port

¼　cup reduced-sodium chicken broth

6　fresh plums, pitted and quartered

　　Fresh rosemary sprigs (optional)

Olive Oil

1. Preheat oven to 300°F. Season pork with kosher salt and pepper. In a 4- to 5-quart oven-going Dutch oven heat oil over medium heat. Add pork; cook for 5 to 8 minutes or until browned, turning roast to brown evenly on all sides. Remove pork from pan; set aside.

2. Add onion and carrot to Dutch oven. Cook about 5 minutes or until the onion is golden brown, stirring frequently. Stir in the rosemary and garlic; cook and stir for 1 minute more. Add port and broth. Return the pork to the pan. Heat just until boiling.

3. Cover Dutch oven and bake for 20 minutes. Add plums to Dutch oven. Bake, covered, for 20 to 25 minutes more or until an instant-read thermometer inserted into center of pork registers 150°F.

4. Transfer the pork to a cutting board; cover with foil and let stand for 15 minutes before slicing. The temperature of the pork after standing should be 160°F. Meanwhile, using a slotted spoon, transfer plums to a serving platter. Place Dutch oven over medium-high heat on the rangetop. Reduce heat; boil gently, uncovered, about 10 minutes or until sauce is reduced to about ¾ cup.

5. To serve, thinly slice pork. Arrange pork slices on platter with plums. Serve with sauce. If desired garnish with fresh rosemary.

Nutrition facts per serving: 367 cal., 10 g total fat (3 g sat. fat), 83 mg chol., 249 mg sodium, 19 g carbo., 2 g fiber, 34 g pro.
Exchanges: 1 Fruit, ½ Other Carbo., 5 Lean Meat, ½ Fat

For Wave 1, this is not appropriate. For Waves 2 and 3, serve with steamed fresh green beans and cooked multigrain pasta.

Wine Pairing: Pinot Noir

CHILI-COATED PORK TENDERLOIN

This fuss-free recipe uses pork tenderloin, the leanest and most tender cut of pork available.
Chili powder and cayenne pepper start heating things up even before it's in the oven.

Prep: 10 minutes **Roast:** 25 minutes **Stand:** 15 minutes **Oven:** 425°F **Makes:** 6 servings

1 tablespoon chili powder

1 teaspoon kosher salt

1 teaspoon dried oregano, crushed

½ teaspoon freshly ground black pepper

½ teaspoon ground cumin

¼ teaspoon cayenne pepper

2 ¾- to 1-pound pork tenderloins

1 recipe Corn and Pepper Relish (optional)

1. Preheat oven to 425°F. For rub, in a small bowl combine chili powder, kosher salt, oregano, black pepper, cumin, and cayenne pepper. Sprinkle rub over all sides of meat; rub in with your fingers.

2. Insert an oven-going meat thermometer into thickest part of one tenderloin. Place meat on a rack in a shallow roasting pan. Roast for 25 to 35 minutes or until thermometer registers 155°F. Cover meat with foil and let stand for 15 minutes before slicing. The temperature of the meat after standing should be 160°F. Slice meat. If desired, serve with Corn and Pepper Relish.

Nutrition facts per serving: 138 cal., 3 g total fat (1 g sat. fat), 73 mg chol., 380 mg sodium, 1 g carbo., 1 g fiber, 24 g pro.
Exchanges: 3½ Very Lean Meat, ½ Fat

Corn and Pepper Relish: In a small bowl combine ¾ cup chopped red bell pepper; ¾ cup loose-pack frozen whole kernel corn, thawed; ⅓ cup chopped red onion; and 3 tablespoons chopped fresh cilantro.

For Wave 1, do not serve with the Corn and Pepper Relish; serve with cooked brown rice and cooked broccoli. For Waves 2 and 3, serve with the Corn and Pepper Relish, cooked brown rice, and fresh nectarine slices.

Wine Pairing: sparkling Pinot Noir

STIR-FRIED PORK AND JICAMA

This is not your typical stir-fry! The intriguing fusion of Mexican and Asian ingredients gives this dish bold flavor and varied texture. If you'd like, prepare the vegetables ahead of time, keeping them covered and chilled for up to 4 hours.

Start to Finish: 30 minutes **Makes:** 4 servings

1 pound lean boneless pork

½ cup cold water

¼ cup dry sherry

¼ cup soy sauce

4 teaspoons cornstarch

1 tablespoon canola oil

1 teaspoon grated fresh ginger

1 clove garlic, minced (½ teaspoon minced)

½ of a medium jicama, peeled and cut into thin bite-size strips (1 cup)

2 medium red and/or green bell peppers, cut into thin bite-size strips

1 green onion, sliced

2 cups shredded fresh spinach or Chinese (napa) cabbage

2 cups hot cooked brown rice

1. Trim fat from pork. If desired, partially freeze pork. Thinly slice pork across grain into bite-size strips. Set aside.

2. For sauce, in a small bowl stir together the water, sherry, soy sauce, and cornstarch. Set aside.

3. Pour canola oil into a wok or large skillet. (Add more oil as necessary during cooking.) Heat over medium-high heat. Stir-fry ginger and garlic in hot oil for 15 seconds. Add jicama, bell pepper strips, and green onion; stir-fry for 1 to 2 minutes or until crisp-tender. Remove vegetables from the wok.

4. Add half of the pork to the hot wok. Stir-fry for 2 to 3 minutes or until cooked through. Remove pork from the wok. Repeat with remaining pork. Return all of the pork to the wok. Push pork from center of the wok.

5. Stir sauce; add sauce to the center of the wok. Cook and stir until thickened and bubbly. Return cooked vegetables to wok; stir to coat all ingredients with sauce. Add spinach. Cook and stir for 1 to 2 minutes more or until heated through. Serve immediately with hot cooked rice.

Nutrition facts per serving: 351 cal., 9 g total fat (2 g sat. fat), 71 mg chol., 1,086 mg sodium, 34 g carbo., 3 g fiber, 29 g pro.
Exchanges: 1½ Vegetable, 1½ Starch, 3½ Very Lean Meat, 2 Fat

For Wave 1, serve with cooked snow pea pods.
For Waves 2 and 3, serve with fresh pineapple.

Wine Pairing: Zinfandel

Spinach   *Bell Peppers*

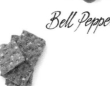

Whole Grains

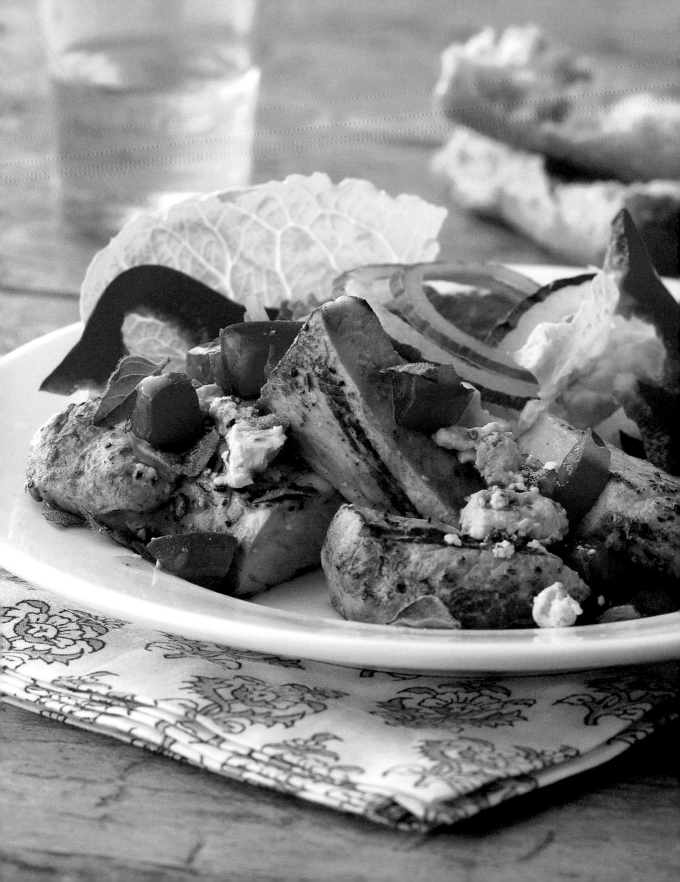

SONOMA express GREEK PORK CHOPS

Balsamic vinegar is aromatic, so a tablespoon is all you need for these chops. The combination of balsamic vinegar, tomatoes, and feta cheese creates a simple but exquisite topping.

Prep: 15 minutes **Grill:** 12 minutes **Makes:** 4 servings

½ cup chopped seeded tomato

1 tablespoon bottled balsamic vinaigrette salad dressing (such as Newman's Own brand)

4 boneless pork loin chops, cut ¾ inch thick (about 1¼ pounds total)

1 teaspoon lemon-pepper seasoning

¼ cup crumbled feta cheese with garlic and herb (1 ounce)

Fresh oregano (optional)

Tomatoes

1. In a small bowl combine tomato and salad dressing; set aside.

2. Trim fat from chops. Sprinkle lemon-pepper seasoning evenly over both sides of each chop. For a charcoal grill, place chops on the rack of an uncovered grill directly over medium coals. Grill for 12 to 15 minutes or until done (160°F) and juices run clear, turning once halfway through grilling. (For a gas grill, preheat grill. Reduce heat to medium. Place chops on grill rack over heat. Cover and grill as above.) Slice pork chops.

3. Transfer pork to four dinner plates. Top chops with feta cheese and tomato mixture. If desired, garnish with oregano.

Nutrition facts per serving: 205 cal., 6 g total fat (2 g sat. fat), 83 mg chol., 646 mg sodium, 2 g carbo., 0 g fiber, 34 g pro.
Exchanges: 4½ Very Lean Meat, 1 Fat

For Wave 1, serve with a mixed green salad and whole grain bread. For Waves 2 and 3, serve with a mixed green salad, whole grain bread, and fresh plum slices.

Wine Pairing: Cabernet Sauvignon

GRILLED SAGE PORK CHOPS

*Sage is an excellent accompaniment to any pork dish. Here it transforms
basic pork chops into an earthy Mediterranean meal.*

Prep: 20 minutes **Grill:** 12 minutes **Makes:** 6 servings

6   boneless pork sirloin chops, cut ¾ inch thick (about 2 pounds total)

Kosher salt

Freshly ground black pepper

4   to 6 cloves garlic, minced (2 to 3 teaspoons minced)

2   tablespoons soy sauce

1   tablespoon chopped fresh sage

1   tablespoon extra-virgin olive oil

2   teaspoons lemon juice

1   tablespoon chopped fresh sage

1   tablespoon chopped fresh flat-leaf parsley

1   tablespoon lemon juice

1   tablespoon extra-virgin olive oil

Olive Oil

1. Trim fat from meat. Season chops with kosher salt and pepper; set aside. For basting sauce, in a small bowl combine garlic, soy sauce, 1 tablespoon sage, 1 tablespoon olive oil, and the 2 teaspoons lemon juice.

2. Brush tops of the chops with half of the basting sauce. For a charcoal grill, place chops on the rack of an uncovered grill directly over medium coals. Grill for 12 to 15 minutes or until done (160°F) and juices run clear, turning and brushing once with the remaining basting sauce halfway through grilling. Discard any remaining basting sauce. (For a gas grill, preheat grill. Reduce heat to medium. Place chops on grill rack over heat. Cover and grill as above.)

3. Meanwhile, in a small bowl combine 1 tablespoon sage, the parsley, the 1 tablespoon lemon juice, and 1 tablespoon olive oil.

4. To serve, cut meat into ¼-inch-thick slices. Top with the parsley mixture.

Nutrition facts per serving: 257 cal., 12 g total fat (3 g sat. fat), 94 mg chol., 489 mg sodium, 2 g carbo., 0 g fiber, 32 g pro.
Exchanges: 4½ Very Lean Meat, 2 Fat

For Wave 1, serve with Mushrooms with Garlic and Herbs (page 209), steamed asparagus, and a whole grain roll. For Waves 2 and 3, serve with Sweet Potato and Cranberry Bake (page 255), fresh pear slices, and a whole grain roll.

Wine Pairing: Pinot Noir

BALSAMIC PORK CHOPS

These pan-fried chops get a touch of tanginess from balsamic vinegar and garlicky onion flavor from the shallot. As one of the smallest members of the onion family, shallots are similar in size to garlic, have cloves like garlic, and even add garlic flavor, but you'll find they still have great sweet onion flavor.

Start to Finish: 25 minutes **Makes:** 4 servings

4   pork loin chops, cut 1 inch thick
    (about 1¾ pounds total)

    Kosher salt

    Freshly ground black pepper

1   tablespoon extra-virgin olive oil

1   medium shallot, minced

½   cup chicken broth

1   tablespoon balsamic vinegar

¼   teaspoon dried thyme, crushed

1   tablespoon chopped flat-leaf parsley

Olive Oil

1. Season meat with kosher salt and pepper. In a very large skillet heat oil over medium heat. Add chops; cook for 8 to 12 minutes or until done (160°F) and juices run clear, turning chops occasionally. (If meat browns too quickly, reduce heat to medium-low.) Transfer to a serving platter; cover and keep warm.

2. Add shallot to skillet, cook and stir for 1 minute. Add broth, vinegar, and thyme. Bring to boiling; reduce heat. Simmer, uncovered, for 2 to 3 minutes or until reduced to about ⅓ cup. Remove from heat. Pour over meat. Sprinkle with parsley.

Nutrition facts per serving: 218 cal., 9 g total fat (3 g sat. fat), 81 mg chol., 319 mg sodium, 2 g carbo., 0 g fiber, 29 g pro.
Exchanges: 4 Very Lean Meat, 1½ Fat

For Wave 1, serve with cooked multigrain pasta and a mixed green salad. For Waves 2 and 3, serve with roasted beets, cooked multigrain pasta, and fresh berries.

Wine Pairing: Pinot Noir

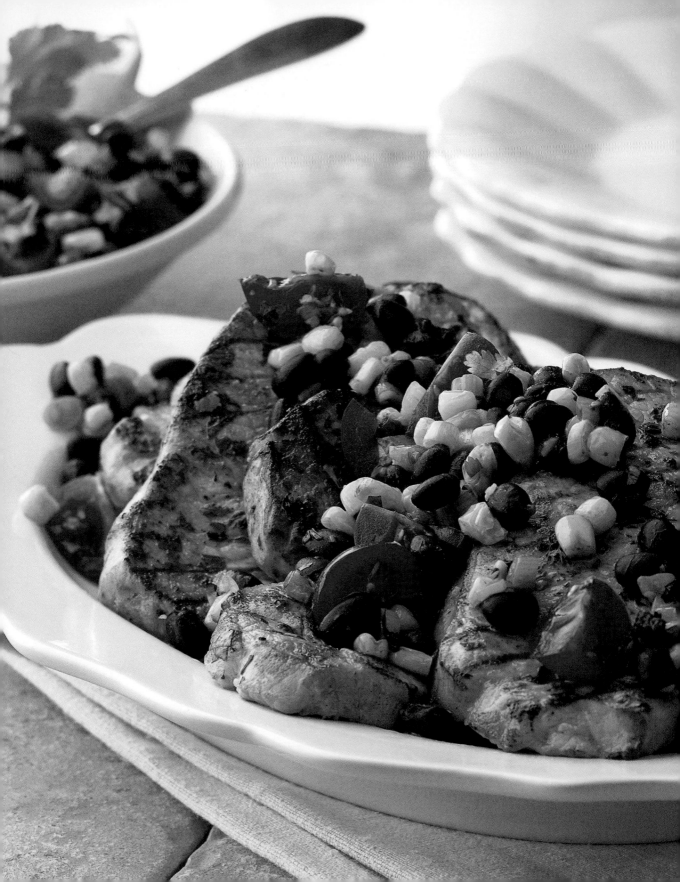

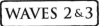
PORK CHOPS WITH SMOKY BLACK BEAN RELISH

These grilled chops have a distinct Southwestern taste. Black beans have a rich, slightly sweet flavor and contain molybdenum, folate, and fiber; they are also rich in antioxidants. When combined with corn, lime, tomatoes, and chile peppers, the result is a truly authentic-tasting meal.

Prep: 25 minutes **Grill:** 7 minutes **Makes:** 6 servings

6 boneless pork top loin chops, cut ½ inch thick (about 1¾ pounds total)

Kosher salt

Freshly ground black pepper

3 tablespoons lime juice

2 tablespoons chopped fresh cilantro

1 tablespoon extra-virgin olive oil

6 cloves garlic, minced (1 tablespoon minced)

1 cup frozen whole kernel corn, thawed

2 cups cherry tomatoes, quartered

1 15-ounce can black beans, rinsed and drained

½ cup sliced green onions

¼ cup chopped fresh cilantro

1 to 2 teaspoons finely chopped canned chipotle chile peppers in adobo sauce*

1. Trim fat from chops. Season chops with kosher salt and pepper. In a small bowl combine 2 tablespoons of the lime juice and 2 tablespoons cilantro; brush over chops.

2. For a charcoal grill, place chops on the rack of an uncovered grill directly over medium coals. Grill for 7 to 9 minutes or until chops are done (160°F) and juices run clear. (For a gas grill preheat grill. Reduce heat to medium. Place chops on grill rack over heat. Cover and grill as above.)

3. Meanwhile, in a large skillet heat oil over medium-high heat. Add garlic; cook for 30 seconds. Add corn; cook and stir about 3 minutes or until lightly browned.

4. In a large bowl combine the corn mixture, tomatoes, black beans, green onions, the ¼ cup cilantro, the chipotle peppers, and the remaining 1 tablespoon lime juice. Season to taste with kosher salt and pepper.

5. Serve chops with corn mixture.

Nutrition facts per serving: 274 cal., 6 g total fat (1 g sat. fat), 78 mg chol., 663 mg sodium, 20 g carbo., 5 g fiber, 38 g pro.
Exchanges: 1 Starch, ½ Other Carbo., 5 Very Lean Meat

*See note, page 76

For Wave 1, this recipe is not appropriate. For Waves 2 and 3, serve with fresh peach slices.

Wine Pairing: Zinfandel

Olive Oil

Tomatoes

PORK WITH MUSHROOMS

This simple combination of pork, mushrooms, and seasonings is the ultimate dish when you're looking for something savory. Buy presliced mushrooms to save on prep time.

Start to Finish: 40 minutes **Makes:** 4 servings

2 tablespoons extra-virgin olive oil

1 pound fresh mushrooms (such as stemmed shiitake, cremini, and/or button), sliced

½ cup finely chopped onion

6 cloves garlic, minced (1 tablespoon minced)

1 tablespoon chopped fresh thyme

½ cup dry white wine

1 tablespoon grated Parmesan cheese

1 tablespoon chopped fresh flat-leaf parsley

¼ teaspoon kosher salt

⅛ teaspoon freshly ground black pepper

4 boneless pork loin chops (about 1¼ pounds total)

Kosher salt

Freshly ground black pepper

1 cup chicken broth

Olive Oil

1. In a large skillet heat 1 tablespoon of the olive oil over medium-high heat. Add mushrooms; cook about 5 minutes or until tender and starting to brown, stirring occasionally. Add onion; cook and stir about 4 minutes or until onion is tender. Add the garlic and thyme; cook and stir for 1 minute. Carefully add wine to skillet. Bring to boiling; reduce heat. Boil gently, uncovered, for 2 to 3 minutes or until most of the liquid has evaporated. Remove from heat; transfer to a medium bowl. Stir in the Parmesan cheese, parsley, the ¼ teaspoon kosher salt, and the ⅛ teaspoon pepper.

2. Season chops lightly with additional kosher salt and pepper. In the same skillet heat the remaining 1 tablespoon oil over medium-high heat. Add chops; cook for 6 minutes, turning once to brown evenly. Add mushroom mixture and broth to skillet around the chops. Bring to boiling; reduce heat. Cover and simmer for 7 to 10 minutes or until pork is done (160°F) and juices run clear. Transfer chops to a serving platter; cover and keep warm.

3. Bring mixture in skillet to boiling; reduce heat; Boil gently, uncovered, for 5 minutes. Spoon some of mushroom mixture over chops; pass remaining mushroom mixture.

Nutrition facts per serving: 334 cal., 11 g total fat (2 g sat. fat), 80 mg chol., 769 mg sodium, 21 g carbo., 3 g fiber, 35 g pro.
Exchanges: ½ Vegetable, 1 Other Carbo., 5 Very Lean Meat, 1½ Fat

For Wave 1, serve with wilted spinach and cooked brown rice. For Waves 2 and 3, serve with cooked brown rice and fresh orange slices.

Wine Pairing: Sauvignon Blanc

BRAISED PORK TENDERLOIN WITH OLIVES AND CAPERS

Olives, capers, and tomatoes, staples of Mediterranean cuisine, contribute a robust, earthy flavor to this tender recipe.

Prep: 35 minutes **Cook:** 15 minutes + 10 minutes **Makes:** 6 servings

2 pounds pork tenderloin

Kosher salt

Freshly ground black pepper

¼ cup extra-virgin olive oil

2 cups 1-inch cubes unpeeled eggplant

2 cups chopped onion

1 cup chopped celery

1 medium red bell pepper, seeded and cut into 1-inch pieces

6 cloves garlic, minced (1 tablespoon minced)

1 14½-ounce can diced tomatoes, undrained

1 cup chicken broth

¼ cup white wine vinegar

¼ cup green olives, pitted and chopped

1 tablespoon capers, rinsed and drained

2 tablespoons chopped fresh mint

2 tablespoons chopped fresh basil

2 tablespoons chopped fresh flat-leaf parsley

1. Trim fat from pork. Cut pork into 1-inch cubes. Season pork with kosher salt and pepper; set aside.

2. In a very large skillet heat 2 tablespoons of the olive oil over medium heat. Add eggplant; cook for 5 minutes, stirring occasionally. Remove eggplant from skillet; set aside.

3. In the same skillet heat 1 tablespoon of the remaining olive oil over medium-high heat. Add pork; cook and stir about 3 minutes or until browned. Remove from skillet; cover and keep warm.

4. Add the remaining 1 tablespoon olive oil to skillet. Add onion, celery, bell pepper, and garlic. Cook and stir for 5 minutes.

5. Stir in undrained tomatoes, chicken broth, vinegar, olives, and capers. Bring to boiling; reduce heat. Simmer, uncovered, about 15 minutes or until most of the liquid is evaporated. Return eggplant and pork to the skillet. Cover and simmer about 10 minutes more or until pork is tender. Stir in mint and basil. Sprinkle with parsley.

Nutrition facts per serving: 326 cal., 15 g total fat (3 g sat. fat), 98 mg chol., 650 mg sodium, 13 g carbo., 4 g fiber, 34 g pro.
Exchanges: 2 Vegetable, 4½ Very Lean Meat, 2½ Fat

For Wave 1, serve with Basil Quinoa with Red Bell Pepper (page 221) and a spinach salad. For Waves 2 and 3, serve with Basil Quinoa with Red Bell Pepper (page 221) and fresh mango slices.

Wine Pairing: Sauvignon Blanc

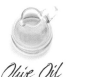

Olive Oil   *Tomatoes*

Bell Peppers

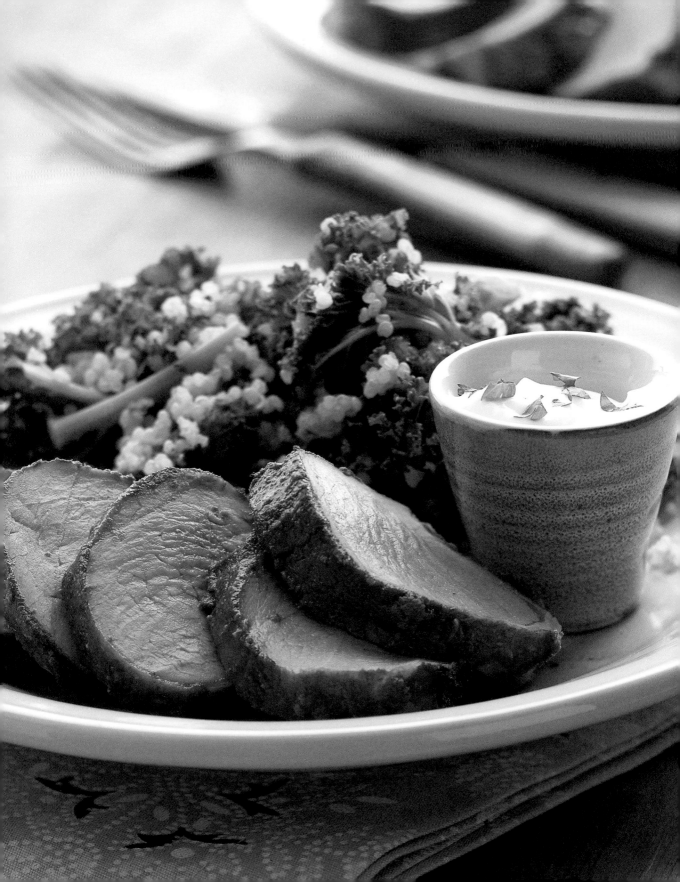

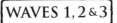
PORK TENDERLOIN WITH QUINOA AND GREENS

Enjoy a roasted pork dinner that's ready in minutes, not hours. If you're having a hard time finding curry paste, check the ethnic section of the grocery store or an Indian or Asian market.

Prep: 20 minutes **Roast:** 25 minutes **Stand:** 15 minutes + 5 minutes **Oven:** 425°F **Makes:** 6 servings

2 tablespoons curry paste*

2 12- to 16-ounce pork tenderloins

2 14-ounce cans chicken broth**

1 cup quinoa*

1 tablespoon extra virgin olive oil

2 cloves garlic, minced (1 teaspoon minced)

12 ounces fresh kale, stemmed and torn

½ cup plain low-fat yogurt (optional)

Chopped fresh flat-leaf parsley (optional)

Nutrition facts per serving: 296 cal., 8 g total fat (2 g sat. fat), 74 mg chol., 468 mg sodium, 27 g carbo., 3 g fiber, 30 g pro.
Exchanges: 1½ Vegetable, 1½ Starch, 3 Very Lean Meat, 1 Fat

*Note: Indian curry paste is available in the ethnic section of many supermarkets. Look for quinoa at a health food store or in the grains section of a large supermarket.

**Note: If you prefer, use reduced-sodium chicken broth.

For Wave 1, serve with Mushrooms with Garlic and Herbs (page 209). For Waves 2 and 3, serve with fresh berries.

Wine Pairing: Chardonnay

1. Preheat oven to 425°F. Using your fingers, rub curry paste on all sides of pork. Place pork on a rack in a shallow roasting pan.

2. Roast pork for 25 to 35 minutes or until an instant-read thermometer inserted in thickest part of tenderloin registers 155°F. Remove pork from oven. Cover with foil and let stand for 15 minutes before slicing. The temperature of the meat after standing should be 160°F.

3. Meanwhile, in a medium saucepan bring 1 can of the broth to boiling over medium-high heat. Add quinoa, olive oil, and garlic; reduce heat. Cover and simmer about 15 minutes or until liquid is absorbed and quinoa is tender. Remove from heat; let stand, covered, for 5 minutes.

4. Meanwhile, in a large saucepan bring the remaining 1 can broth and the kale to boiling over medium-high heat; reduce heat. Cover and simmer about 20 minutes or until kale is tender, stirring occasionally. Using a slotted spoon, transfer kale to a large serving bowl; stir in quinoa.

5. Thinly slice pork. Serve with quinoa mixture and, if desired, yogurt. If desired, garnish with parsley.

Olive Oil

Whole Grains

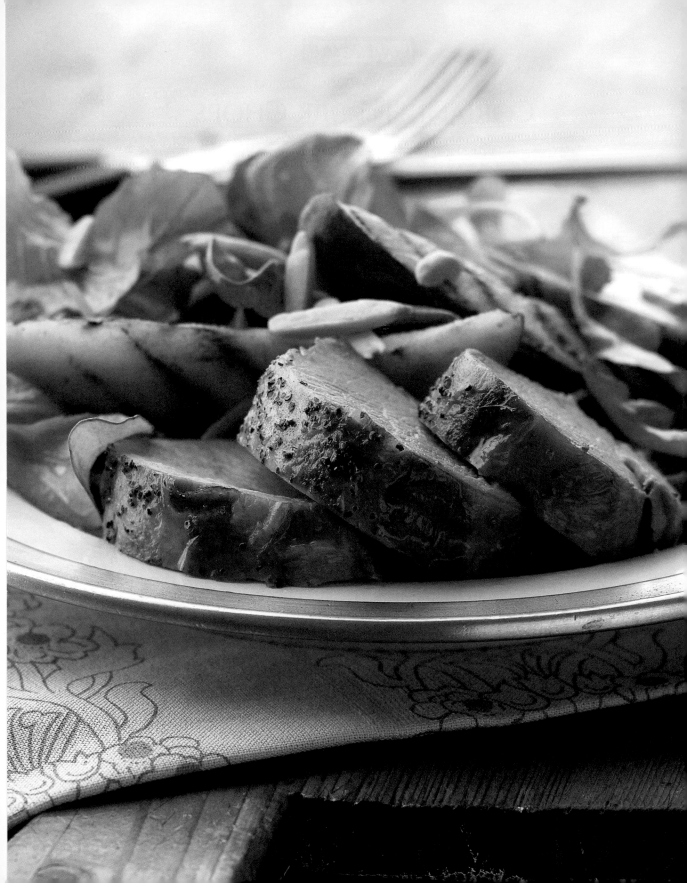

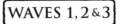
GRILLED PORK WITH GRILLED PEARS, ARUGULA, AND TOASTED ALMONDS

Almond accents add crunch, calcium, fiber, and riboflavin to this luscious pork and pear combo. A simple vinaigrette dresses the fruit and greens with delicate flavor.

Prep: 25 minutes **Grill:** 30 minutes + 5 minutes **Stand:** 15 minutes **Makes:** 4 servings

1 1-pound pork tenderloin

Kosher salt

Freshly ground black pepper

2 tablespoons extra-virgin olive oil

2 tablespoons lemon juice

2 medium pears, cored and each cut into 8 wedges

2 teaspoons lemon juice

4 cups torn arugula leaves or fresh baby spinach

2 cups fresh baby spinach

2 tablespoons slivered almonds, toasted

Olive Oil

Spinach

Almonds

1. Trim fat from meat. Season meat with kosher salt and pepper. For a charcoal grill, arrange hot coals around a drip pan. Test for medium-hot heat above the pan. Place meat on grill rack over drip pan. Cover and grill for 30 to 35 minutes or until an instant-read thermometer inserted in center of meat registers 155°F. (For a gas grill, preheat grill. Reduce heat to medium high. Adjust for indirect cooking. Place meat on grill rack. Cover and grill as above.) Remove meat from grill. Cover with foil and let stand for 15 minutes before slicing. The temperature of the meat after standing should be 160°F.

2. Meanwhile, for vinaigrette, in a small bowl whisk together olive oil and the 2 tablespoons lemon juice; set aside. In a medium bowl toss pear wedges with the 2 teaspoons lemon juice.

3. Remove meat from grill; let stand for 10 minutes before slicing. While the meat stands, add pear wedges to grill rack directly over the coals. Grill, uncovered, about 5 minutes or just until pears are tender and warmed through, turning to brown evenly.

4. In a large bowl combine arugula, spinach, pear wedges, and almonds. Add the vinaigrette and toss to coat. Season to taste with additional kosher salt and pepper. Thinly slice pork. Serve with the arugula-pear mixture.

Nutrition facts per serving: 275 cal., 12 g total fat (2 g sat. fat), 73 mg chol., 184 mg sodium, 16 g carbo., 4 g fiber, 26 g pro.
Exchanges: 1½ Vegetable, ½ Fruit, 3 Very Lean Meat, 2 Fat

For Wave 1, omit the pears and serve with a whole grain roll. For Waves 2 and 3, serve with a whole grain roll.

Wine Pairing: Sauvignon Blanc

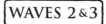

PORK CHOPS WITH PORT AND CRANBERRIES

Sophisticated and elegant, this recipe has immense flavor but is amazingly simple
The ruby-color sauce is wonderfully tart and full of antioxidants.

Start to Finish: 25 minutes **Makes:** 4 servings

1 cup chicken broth or reduced-sodium chicken broth

½ cup port

½ teaspoon grated fresh ginger

½ cup fresh cranberries

2 teaspoons lemon juice

1 tablespoon chicken broth or reduced-sodium chicken broth

½ teaspoon cornstarch

   Kosher salt

   Freshly ground black pepper

4 boneless pork sirloin chops, cut ¾ inch thick (about 1½ pounds total)

1 tablespoon chopped fresh rosemary

1 tablespoon extra-virgin olive oil

Olive Oil

1. In a small saucepan combine the 1 cup chicken broth, the port, and ginger. Bring to boiling. Boil gently for 15 to 20 minutes or until liquid is reduced to ½ cup. Add cranberries; cook just until cranberries begin to pop. Stir in lemon juice. In a small bowl stir together the 1 tablespoon chicken broth and the cornstarch; add to the cranberry mixture. Cook and stir until thickened and bubbly; cook and stir for 2 minutes more. Season to taste with kosher salt and pepper.

2. Meanwhile, season pork chops with kosher salt and pepper. Sprinkle chops evenly with rosemary, pressing in lightly with fingers. In a large skillet heat olive oil over medium-high heat. Add pork chops; cook for 8 to 12 minutes or until chops are done (160°F) and juices run clear, turning once. Serve chops with cranberry mixture.

Nutrition facts per serving: 305 cal., 10 g total fat (3 g sat. fat), 107 mg chol., 386 mg sodium, 7 g carbo., 1 g fiber, 36 g pro.
Exchanges: ½ Other Carbo., 5 Very Lean Meat, 2 Fat

For Wave 1, this is not appropriate. For Waves 2 and 3, serve with fresh pear slices, cooked multigrain pasta, and cooked zucchini.

Wine Pairing: Cabernet Sauvignon

SPICE-RUBBED PORK CHOPS

A conglomeration of full-flavored spices guarantees that these chops will be red hot!

Prep: 15 minutes **Marinate:** 4 to 6 hours **Grill:** 11 minutes **Makes:** 4 servings

4   pork rib chops, cut ¾ inch thick
    (about 1½ pounds total)

¼   cup lime juice

1   tablespoon chili powder

1   tablespoon extra-virgin olive oil

2   cloves garlic, minced (1 teaspoon minced)

2   teaspoons ground cumin

1   teaspoon ground cinnamon

½   teaspoon bottled hot pepper sauce

¼   teaspoon kosher salt

Olive Oil

1. Trim fat from chops. Place chops in a self-sealing plastic bag set in a shallow dish. For marinade, in a small bowl stir together lime juice, chili powder, olive oil, garlic, cumin, cinnamon, hot pepper sauce, and kosher salt; pour over chops. Seal bag; turn to coat chops. Marinate in the refrigerator for 4 to 6 hours, turning bag occasionally.

2. Drain chops, discarding marinade. For a charcoal grill, place chops on the rack of an uncovered grill directly over medium coals. Grill for 11 to 14 minutes or until pork is done (160°F) and juices run clear, turning once. (For a gas grill, preheat grill. Reduce heat to medium. Place chops on grill rack over heat. Cover and grill as above.)

Nutrition facts per serving: 259 cal., 11 g total fat (3 g sat. fat), 106 mg chol., 150 mg sodium, 2 g carbo., 1 g fiber, 36 g pro.
Exchanges: 5 Very Lean Meat, 2 Fat

For Wave 1, serve with cooked quinoa and cooked asparagus and red bell peppers. For Waves 2 and 3, serve with Spicy Black-Eyed Pea Salad (page 216) and fresh tangerine slices.

Wine Pairing: sparkling semisweet or rosé

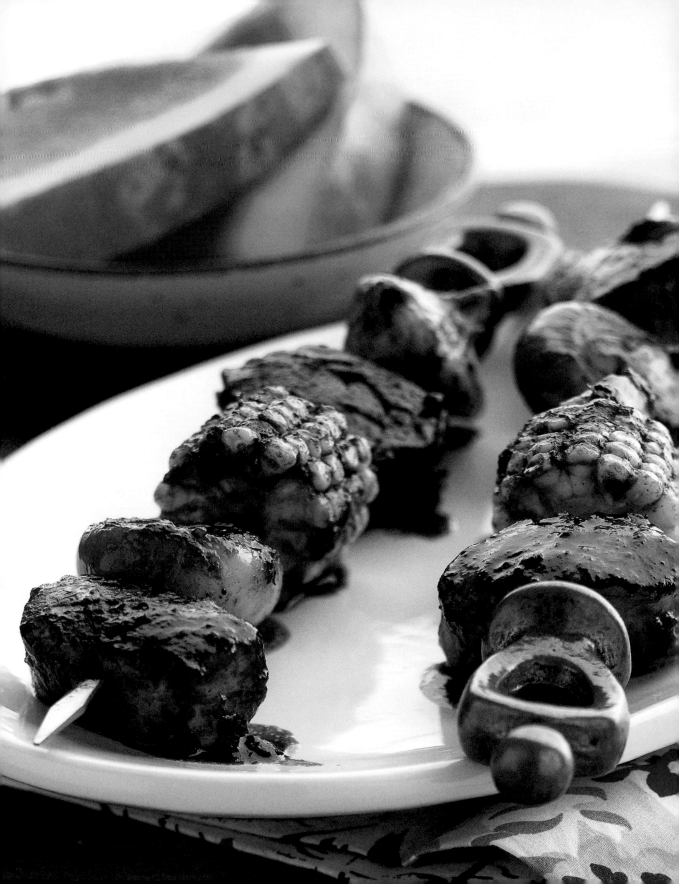

SONOMA express JAMAICAN PORK KABOBS

An island air provided by mango chutney and Pickapeppa sauce makes this pork dish excellent summer fare. Pickapeppa, Jamaica's renowned condiment, has a sweet, slightly spicy flavor and can usually be found with the other condiments at grocery stores.

Prep: 15 minutes **Grill:** 12 minutes **Makes:** 4 servings

2 ears of corn, husked and cleaned

1 12- to 14-ounce pork tenderloin

1 small red onion, cut into ½-inch-thick slices or thin wedges

16 baby pattypan squash (each about 1 inch in diameter) or 4 tomatillos, quartered

¼ cup mango chutney, finely chopped

3 tablespoons Pickapeppa sauce

1 tablespoon canola oil

1 tablespoon water

1. Cut corn crosswise into 1-inch pieces. In a medium saucepan cook corn pieces in a small amount of boiling water for 3 minutes; drain and rinse with cold water. Meanwhile, cut pork tenderloin into 1½-inch pieces. On long metal skewers, alternately thread tenderloin, onion, squash or tomatillos, and corn pieces, leaving a ¼ inch space between pieces.

2. In a small bowl combine chutney, Pickapeppa sauce, canola oil, and the water; set aside.

3. For a charcoal grill, place skewers on the rack of an uncovered grill directly over medium coals. Grill for 12 to 14 minutes or until pork is done and vegetables are tender, turning once halfway through grilling and brushing with the chutney mixture during the last 5 minutes of grilling. (For a gas grill, preheat grill. Reduce heat to medium. Place meat on the grill rack over heat. Cover and grill as above.)

Nutrition facts per serving: 219 cal., 7 g total fat (1 g sat. fat), 55 mg chol., 173 mg sodium, 21 g carbo., 2 g fiber, 20 g pro.
Exchanges: 1 Vegetable, ½ Starch, ½ Other Carbo., 2½ Very Lean Meat, 1 Fat

For Wave 1, this is not appropriate. For Waves 2 and 3, serve with watermelon and cooked quinoa.

Wine Pairing: sparkling semisweet or rosé

CATALONIAN PORK CHOPS WITH PLUMS

Pork dishes are popular in Spain's Catalan cuisine. This one combines sweet, juicy plums, which contain vitamin C and other antioxidants, with the salty and savory flavors of pork.

Start to Finish: 30 minutes **Makes:** 4 servings

4 boneless pork loin chops (1¼ to 1½ pounds total)

Kosher salt

Freshly ground black pepper

1 tablespoon extra-virgin olive oil

½ cup dry red wine

½ cup water

1 3-inch-long cinnamon stick

4 plums, pitted and cut into thick wedges

Olive Oil

1. Season pork chops with kosher salt and pepper. In a large skillet heat oil over medium-high heat. Add pork chops; reduce heat to medium and cook for 8 to 12 minutes or until slightly pink in the center (160°F), turning once halfway through cooking. Remove chops from skillet; cover and keep warm.

2. For plum sauce, carefully add wine to skillet, stirring to lift up any browned bits. Add the water and cinnamon stick. Bring to boiling. Boil gently, uncovered, about 5 minutes or until reduced by half.

3. Add plums to skillet; cook, covered, for 3 to 5 minutes or just until plums are tender. Season to taste with kosher salt and pepper. Discard cinnamon stick. Serve plum sauce with pork.

Nutrition facts per serving: 249 cal., 6 g total fat (1 g sat. fat), 78 mg chol., 359 mg sodium, 8 g carbo., 1 g fiber, 32 g pro.
Exchanges: ½ Fruit, 4½ Very Lean Meat, 1½ Fat

For Wave 1, this is not appropriate. For Waves 2 and 3, serve with Barley Risotto with Roasted Squash (page 192).

Wine Pairing: Zinfandel

FAJITA CHOPS

A colorful mélange of mango, tomato, and Great Northern beans sets the stage for delicious grilled or broiled pork slices. Don't have any Great Northern beans on hand? Any variety of white bean will work in this recipe.

Prep: 20 minutes **Broil:** 9 minutes **Stand:** 30 minutes **Makes:** 4 servings

1   lime
1   15-ounce can Great Northern beans, rinsed and drained
1   large mango, pitted, peeled, and chopped, or 2 medium nectarines or peaches, peeled, pitted, and chopped
1   small roma tomato, seeded and chopped
¼   cup sliced green onions
2   tablespoons cider vinegar
1   tablespoon finely chopped fresh jalapeño chile pepper*
1   teaspoon honey
½   teaspoon fajita seasoning
2   cloves garlic, minced (1 teaspoon minced)
4   boneless pork loin chops, cut ¾ inch thick (about 1½ pounds total)
1   teaspoon fajita seasoning
    Lime wedges (optional)

1. Finely shred ½ teaspoon peel from the lime. Squeeze juice from lime. Reserve 2 teaspoons of the lime juice to brush on the pork chops.

2. For salad, in a medium bowl combine finely shredded lime peel, remaining lime juice, beans, mango, tomato, green onions, vinegar, chile pepper, honey, the ½ teaspoon fajita seasoning, and the garlic. Let stand at room temperature for 30 minutes, stirring occasionally. (Or cover and refrigerate for up to 24 hours.)

3. Trim fat from chops. Brush both sides of each chop with the reserved 2 teaspoons lime juice. Sprinkle chops with the 1 teaspoon fajita seasoning.

4. Preheat broiler. Place chops on the unheated rack of a broiler pan. Broil 3 to 4 inches from the heat for 9 to 11 minutes or until pork is done (160°F) and juices run clear, turning once. Slice chops and serve with salad. If desired, serve with lime wedges.

Nutrition facts per serving: 433 cal., 13 g total fat (5 g sat. fat), 107 mg chol., 185 mg sodium, 37 g carbo., 7 g fiber, 41 g pro.
Exchanges: ½ Vegetable, ½ Fruit, 1½ Starch, 5 Lean Meat

Grilling directions: For a charcoal grill, place chops on the rack of an uncovered grill directly over medium coals. Grill for 12 to 15 minutes or until done (160°F) and juices run clear, turning once. (For a gas grill, preheat grill. Reduce heat to medium. Place chops on grill rack over heat. Cover and grill as above.)

*See note, page 76

For Wave 1, this is not appropriate. For Waves 2 and 3, serve with cooked green beans.

Wine Pairing: Zinfandel

Tomatoes

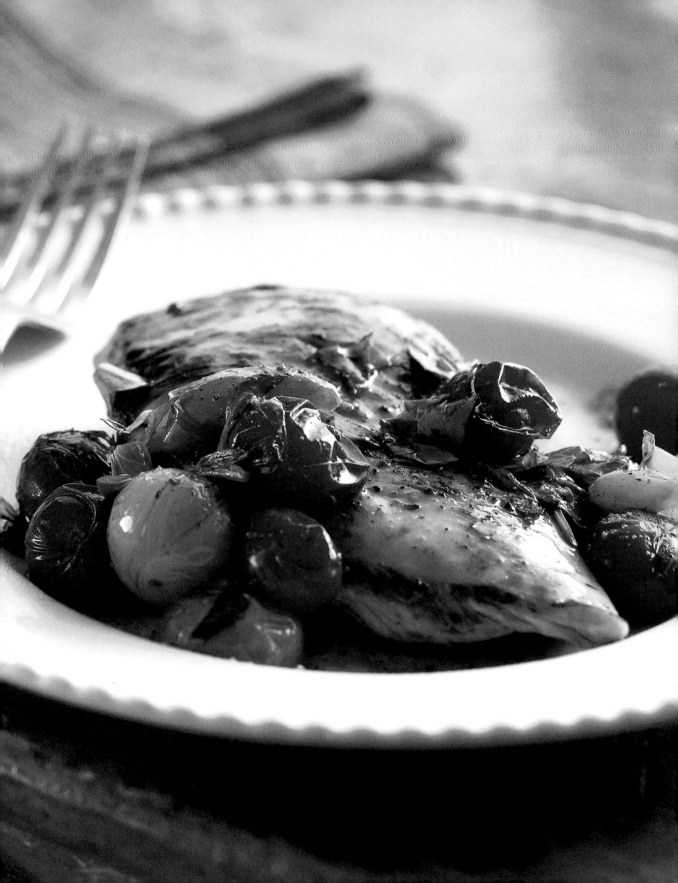

Chicken & Turkey

These recipes use favorite Sonoma ingredients to create new taste experiences with chicken and turkey. Basil, ginger, pepper, cilantro, garlic, mint, and turmeric are just some of the many spices that bring a wine country taste to your table. What better way to expand your chicken repertoire?

SAUTÉED CHICKEN WITH MARSALA

*This version of the classic chicken dish is braised with Marsala wine,
prosciutto, and a mixture of seasonings.*

Start to Finish: 35 minutes   **Makes:** 4 servings

4   skinless, boneless chicken breast halves
    (1 to 1¼ pounds total)

¼   teaspoon kosher salt

⅛   teaspoon freshly ground black pepper

1   tablespoon extra-virgin olive oil

1   tablespoon finely chopped proscuitto

4   cloves garlic, minced (2 teaspoons
    minced)

¾   cup dry Marsala

1   cup chicken broth

2   tablespoons capers, rinsed, drained,
    and chopped

2   tablespoons chopped fresh
    flat-leaf parsley

2   teaspoons chopped fresh sage

Olive Oil

1. Season chicken with kosher salt and pepper.
In a large skillet heat 2 teaspoons of the olive
oil over medium heat. Add chicken; cook for
8 to 10 minutes or until tender and no longer
pink (170°F), turning once. Transfer to a serving
platter; cover and keep warm.

2. In the same skillet combine the remaining
1 teaspoon olive oil, the proscuitto, and garlic.
Cook for 2 minutes, stirring occasionally. Add
Marsala. Bring just to boiling; reduce heat.
Simmer, uncovered, for 4 to 5 minutes or until
reduced to ¼ cup. Add chicken broth, capers,
parsley, and sage. Return to boiling; boil gently
about 8 minutes or until reduced to ⅔ cup. Return
chicken to skillet; heat through.

Nutrition facts per serving: 205 cal., 5 g total fat
(1 g sat. fat), 67 mg chol., 577 mg sodium, 3 g carbo.,
0 g fiber, 27 g pro.
Exchanges: 4 Very Lean Meat, 1 Fat

*For Wave 1, serve with cooked multigrain pasta
and wilted spinach. For Waves 2 and 3, serve
with cooked multigrain pasta, wilted spinach,
and fresh berries.*

Wine Pairing: Sauvignon Blanc

INDIAN-STYLE CURRIED CHICKEN

Indian dishes commonly feature many aromatic spices such as ginger, cumin, turmeric, and coriander. These spices combine in this dish to bring a slightly exotic flavor to this saucy chicken.

Prep: 30 minutes **Cook:** 10 minutes + 15 minutes **Makes:** 4 servings

1 pound skinless, boneless chicken breast halves, cut into 1-inch pieces

1 tablespoon lemon juice

½ teaspoon kosher salt

¼ teaspoon freshly ground black pepper

3 medium tomatoes, cored and quartered

3 tablespoons coarsely chopped garlic

1 tablespoon coarsely chopped fresh ginger

2 tablespoons extra-virgin olive oil

2 cups finely chopped onion

2 teaspoons ground coriander

½ teaspoon ground cumin

¼ teaspoon cayenne pepper

¼ teaspoon ground turmeric

¼ cup chopped fresh cilantro

½ teaspoon garam masala

2 cups hot cooked brown basmati or long grain brown rice

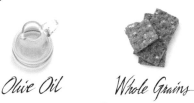

Olive Oil   *Whole Grains*

Tomatoes

1. Place chicken in a medium bowl. Add lemon juice, kosher salt, and black pepper; toss to coat. Set aside.

2. In a blender or food processor combine tomatoes, garlic, and ginger. Cover and blend or process until smooth, stopping and scraping side as necessary; set aside.

3. In a large skillet heat olive oil over medium heat. Add onion; cook and stir about 8 minutes or until golden brown. Add tomato mixture, coriander, cumin, cayenne pepper, and turmeric. Bring to boiling; reduce heat. Simmer, uncovered, for 10 minutes, stirring occasionally.

4. Add chicken to the skillet; stir to coat with the tomato mixture. Return to boiling; reduce heat. Cover and simmer about 15 minutes or until chicken is tender and no longer pink. Remove from the heat; stir in cilantro and garam masala.

5. Serve with brown rice.

Nutrition facts per serving: 362 cal., 10 g total fat (2 g sat. fat), 66 mg chol., 317 mg sodium, 38 g carbo., 5 g fiber, 31 g pro.
Exchanges: 1 Vegetable, 2 Starch, 3½ Very Lean Meat, 1½ Fat

For Wave 1, serve with cooked zucchini and a tossed green salad. For Waves 2 and 3, serve with a tossed green salad and fresh pineapple.

Wine Pairing: sparkling semisweet

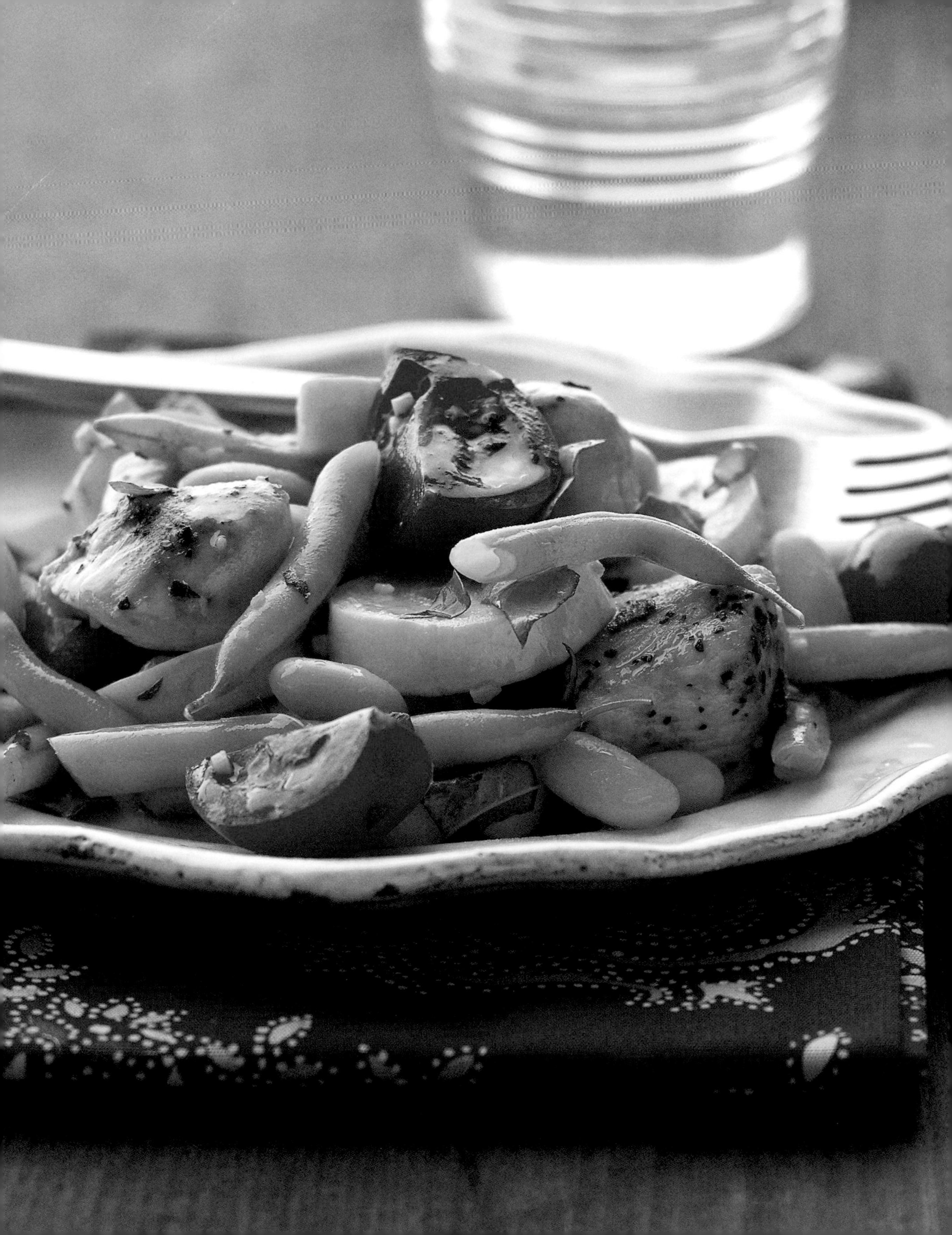

SUMMER VEGETABLE CHICKEN SAUTÉ

Submerging the green beans in ice water immediately after blanching them helps the beans maintain their color and crispness by halting the cooking process until you're ready to finish the recipe.

Start to Finish: 40 minutes **Makes:** 4 servings

2 cups fresh green beans, cut into 2-inch-long pieces

1 tablespoon extra-virgin olive oil

1 pound skinless, boneless chicken breast halves, cut into 1-inch pieces

1 tablespoon chopped fresh oregano or thyme

2 cups sliced yellow summer squash and/or zucchini

1 15-ounce can cannellini beans (white kidney beans), rinsed and drained

¼ cup reduced-sodium chicken broth

6 cloves garlic, minced (1 tablespoon minced)

1 cup cherry tomatoes, halved

1 tablespoon chopped fresh basil or flat-leaf parsley

¼ teaspoon kosher salt

¼ teaspoon freshly ground black pepper

1. In a covered medium saucepan cook green beans in a small amount of salted boiling water for 8 to 10 minutes or until crisp-tender. Drain; submerse beans in enough ice water to cover and let stand until cool. Drain again; set aside.

2. Meanwhile, in a very large skillet heat olive oil over medium heat. In a large bowl toss chicken with oregano. Add chicken to hot oil in skillet, cook for 5 to 6 minutes or until no longer pink, stirring frequently. Remove chicken from skillet and set aside.

3. Add squash to the skillet; cook and stir over medium-high heat for 3 minutes. Stir in chicken, green beans, cannellini beans, chicken broth, and garlic. Bring to boiling. Add tomatoes, basil, kosher salt, and pepper. Cook about 1 minute or until heated through.

Nutrition facts per serving: 257 cal., 5 g total fat (1 g sat. fat), 66 mg chol., 388 mg sodium, 24 g carbo., 8 g fiber, 35 g pro.
Exchanges: 1½ Vegetable, 1 Starch, 3½ Very Lean Meat, ½ Fat

For Wave 1, serve with a tossed green salad. For Waves 2 and 3, serve with fresh apple slices.

Wine Pairing: Sauvignon Blanc

Olive Oil

Tomatoes

CHICKEN WITH TARRAGON

High amounts of tarragon, onion, and sherry vinegar ensure tremendous flavor. Commonly used in classic French dishes, tarragon is earthy and minty with a licoricelike flavor.

Prep: 30 minutes **Cook:** 15 minutes + 10 minutes **Makes:** 4 servings

4   skinless, boneless chicken breast halves (1 to 1¼ pounds total)

    Kosher salt

    Freshly ground black pepper

1   tablespoon extra-virgin olive oil

16   pearl onions, peeled (about 8 ounces)

1   cup thinly sliced onion

8   cloves garlic, peeled

2   sprigs fresh thyme

1   bay leaf

6   tablespoons sherry vinegar

1   tablespoon tomato paste

1   tablespoon Dijon-style mustard

1½   cups reduced-sodium chicken broth or chicken stock

2   to 3 tablespoons chopped fresh tarragon

2   cups hot cooked multigrain pasta (such as Barilla Plus) (optional)

1. Season chicken with kosher salt and pepper. In a large skillet heat olive oil over medium heat. Add chicken; cook for 4 to 6 minutes or until browned, turning once. Remove chicken from skillet. Set aside.

2. Add the pearl onions, sliced onion, garlic cloves, thyme, and bay leaf to the skillet. Cover and cook over low heat for 5 minutes. Add half of the sherry vinegar. Place the chicken on top of the onion mixture. Cover and cook over low heat for 15 to 20 minutes or until chicken is tender and no longer pink (170°F). Remove chicken from the skillet; cover and keep warm.

3. Add remaining sherry vinegar to skillet; cook, uncovered, about 3 minutes or until reduced to a syrup consistency. Stir in the tomato paste and mustard. Add the chicken broth. Bring to boiling; reduce heat. Simmer, uncovered, about 10 minutes or until sauce is reduced to 2 to 2½ cups. Discard bay leaf. Stir in the tarragon. Season to taste with kosher salt and pepper.

4. To serve, place chicken on a serving platter. Spoon sauce and onions over chicken. If desired, serve with hot cooked pasta.

Nutrition facts per serving: 228 cal., 5 g total fat (1 g sat. fat), 66 mg chol., 521 mg sodium, 15 g carbo., 2 g fiber, 30 g pro.
Exchanges: 1½ Vegetable, 4 Very Lean Meat, 1 Fat

For Wave 1, serve with steamed broccoli. For Waves 2 and 3, serve with fresh grapes.

Wine Pairing: Sauvignon Blanc

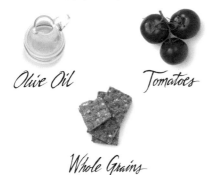

Olive Oil   *Tomatoes*

Whole Grains

SONOMA express ITALIAN-STYLE CHICKEN CUTLETS

This recipe for pan-fried cutlets is quick and easy. The blend of bread crumbs, parsley, rosemary, and Parmesan creates an Italian-flavored crust around the chicken

Prep: 15 minutes **Cook:** 10 minutes **Makes:** 4 servings

4 skinless, boneless chicken breast halves (1 to 1½ pounds total)

¼ teaspoon kosher salt

¼ teaspoon freshly ground black pepper

¾ cup fine dry whole wheat bread crumbs

2 tablespoons freshly grated Parmesan cheese

1 tablespoon chopped fresh flat-leaf parsley

1 teaspoon chopped fresh rosemary

1 egg

1 egg white

2 tablespoons extra-virgin olive oil

Lemon wedges (optional)

Olive Oil

Whole Grains

1. Place each chicken piece between 2 pieces of plastic wrap. Using the flat side of a meat mallet, pound chicken lightly until ½-inch thickness. Remove plastic wrap. Season chicken with kosher salt and pepper.

2. In a shallow dish combine bread crumbs, Parmesan cheese, parsley, and rosemary. Place whole egg and egg white in another shallow dish; beat slightly. Dip chicken in beaten egg, then coat with crumb mixture.

3. In a large skillet heat olive oil over medium-high heat. Add chicken and cook for 10 to 12 minutes or until chicken is no longer pink, turning once. If desired, serve chicken with lemon wedges.

Nutrition facts per serving: 264 cal., 11 g total fat (2 g sat. fat), 121 mg chol., 349 mg sodium, 9 g carbo., 1 g fiber, 31 g pro.
Exchanges: ½ Starch, 4 Very Lean Meat, 2 Fat

For Wave 1, serve with cooked multigrain pasta, a tossed green salad, and Ratatouille Niçoise (page 269). For Waves 2 and 3, serve with cooked multigrain pasta, Ratatouille Niçoise (page 269), and fresh grapes.

Wine Pairing: sparkling semisweet

INDIAN-SPICED CHICKEN WITH VEGETABLES

The ingredient list looks extensive, but the recipe makes both a full flavored marinade and an accompanying salads. Don't worry, many of the ingredients are spices you'll already have on hand.

Prep: 30 minutes **Marinate:** 30 minutes to 4 hours **Grill:** 6 minutes **Makes:** 4 servings

1 pound skinless, boneless chicken breast halves

½ cup plain low-fat yogurt

2 tablespoons chopped fresh flat-leaf parsley

1 tablespoon ground coriander

1 tablespoon grated fresh ginger

2 teaspoons finely chopped fresh jalapeño chile pepper*

1 clove garlic, minced (½ teaspoon minced)

¼ teaspoon kosher salt

½ teaspoon ground cumin

¼ teaspoon ground cardamom

⅛ teaspoon freshly ground black pepper

3 cups fresh baby spinach leaves

1 large red or green bell pepper, seeded and thinly sliced

½ cup thinly sliced red onion

3 tablespoons chopped fresh cilantro

3 tablespoons lemon juice

2 tablespoon extra-virgin olive oil

¼ teaspoon kosher salt

⅛ teaspoon freshly ground black pepper

1. Cut chicken into 1-inch pieces. Set aside.

2. In a medium bowl combine yogurt, parsley, coriander, ginger, chile pepper, garlic, ¼ teaspoon kosher salt, the cumin, cardamom, and ⅛ teaspoon black pepper. Add the chicken; toss gently to coat. Cover and marinate in the refrigerator for 30 minutes to 4 hours.

3. Meanwhile, in a large bowl combine spinach, bell pepper, red onion, cilantro, lemon juice, olive oil, the ¼ teaspoon kosher salt, and ⅛ teaspoon black pepper. Set aside.

4. Thread chicken onto eight skewers,** leaving a ¼-inch space between pieces. For a charcoal grill, place skewers on the greased rack of an uncovered grill directly over medium-hot coals. Grill about 6 minutes or until no longer pink, turning skewers to brown chicken evenly. (For a gas grill, preheat grill. Reduce heat to medium-high. Place skewers on the greased grill rack over heat. Cover and grill as above.)

5. Serve chicken skewers with spinach mixture.

Nutrition facts per serving: 236 cal., 9 g total fat (2 g sat. fat), 68 mg chol., 706 mg sodium, 9 g carbo., 2 g fiber, 30 g pro.
Exchanges: 1½ Vegetable, 4 Very Lean Meat, 1½ Fat

*See note, page 76

**Note: If using wooden skewers, soak in enough water to cover for at least 1 hour before serving.

For Wave 1, serve with whole wheat pita wedges. For Waves 2 and 3, serve with whole wheat pita wedges and fresh mango slices.

Wine Pairing: sparkling semisweet

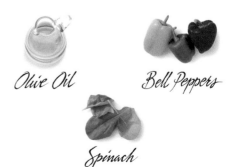

Olive Oil *Bell Peppers*

Spinach

CHICKEN WITH ROQUEFORT

Draped in a decadent sauce, this combination of grilled pears and chicken gets a full, rich flavor from Roquefort cheese. Ready in less than 30 minutes, this dish only appears elaborate.

Prep: 15 minutes **Grill:** 5 minutes + 7 minutes **Makes:** 4 servings

½ cup fat-free plain yogurt

¼ cup chopped red onion

2 tablespoons crumbled Roquefort or blue cheese

1 tablespoon chopped fresh chives

⅛ teaspoon ground white pepper

2 small pears, halved lengthwise, cored, and stemmed

Lemon juice

4 skinless, boneless chicken breast halves (1 to 1¼ pounds total)

Kosher salt

Freshly ground black pepper

1. For sauce, in a small bowl combine yogurt, red onion, Roquefort cheese, chives, and white pepper. Cover and chill until ready to serve. Brush cut sides of pears with lemon juice. Set aside.

2. Season chicken with kosher salt and black pepper. For a charcoal grill, place chicken on the rack of an uncovered grill directly over medium coals. Grill for 5 minutes. Turn chicken. Place pears on grill, cut sides down. Grill chicken and pears for 7 to 10 minutes or until chicken is tender and no longer pink (170°F). (For a gas grill, preheat grill. Reduce heat to medium. Place chicken, then pears on grill rack over heat. Cover and grill as above.)

3. Serve chicken and pears with sauce.

Nutrition facts per serving: 199 cal., 5 g total fat (2 g sat. fat), 63 mg chol., 168 mg sodium, 14 g carbo., 2 g fiber, 25 g pro.
Exchanges: 1 Fruit, 3½ Very Lean Meat, ½ Fat

For Wave 1, omit the pears and serve with a mixed green salad, Wine Country Grain Medley (page 220), and Mushrooms with Garlic and Herbs (page 209). For Waves 2 and 3, serve with Brown Rice Pilaf (page 217) and Mushrooms with Garlic and Herbs (page 209).

Wine Pairing: Chardonnay

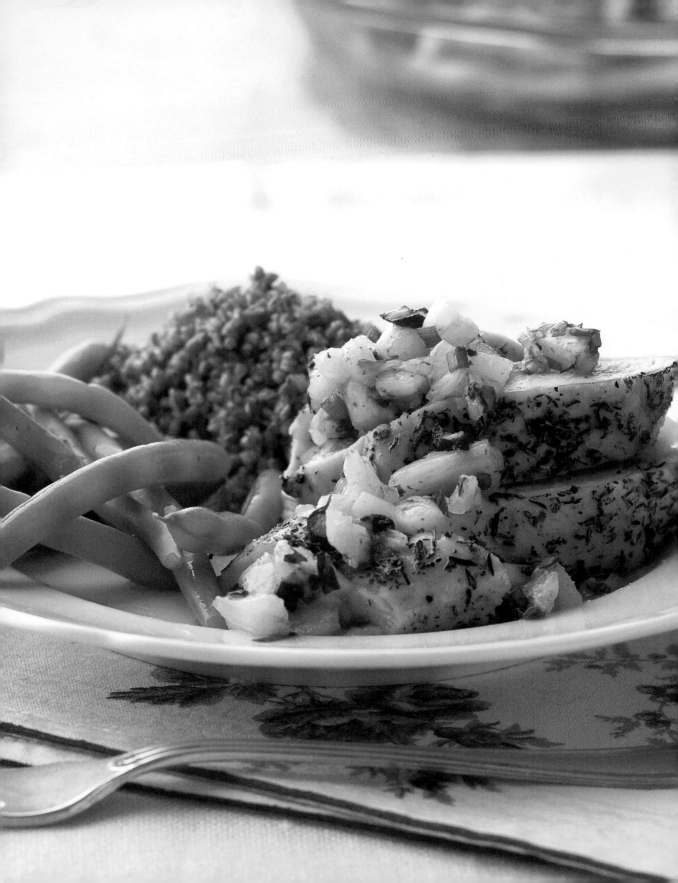

CHICKEN WITH FRUIT SALSA

These juicy chicken breasts are paired with a sweet and fiery salsa that's exploding with flavor. Chipotle peppers give the salsa a spicy kick, so if you like it hot, use the high end of the range.

Prep: 20 minutes **Broil:** 12 minutes **Stand:** 30 minutes **Makes:** 4 servings

1½ cups chopped fresh pineapple

1 to 2 canned chipotle chile peppers in adobo sauce, drained, seeded, and finely chopped*

2 tablespoons chopped fresh chives

1 tablespoon honey

1 teaspoon finely shredded lime peel or lemon peel

2 teaspoons lime juice or lemon juice

4 skinless, boneless chicken breast halves (1 to 1¼ pounds total)

1 teaspoon extra-virgin olive oil

1 teaspoon dried thyme, crushed

¼ teaspoon kosher salt

¼ teaspoon freshly ground black pepper

Olive Oil

1. Preheat broiler. For salsa, in a medium bowl stir together pineapple, chile peppers, chives, honey, lime peel, and lime juice. Let stand at room temperature for 30 minutes.

2. Meanwhile, lightly brush chicken with olive oil. In a small bowl stir together thyme, kosher salt, and black pepper. Sprinkle evenly over chicken; rub in with your fingers.

3. Place chicken on the unheated rack of broiler pan. Broil 4 to 5 inches from heat for 12 to 15 minutes or until chicken is tender and no longer pink (170°F), turning once.

4. Slice chicken and serve with salsa.

Nutrition facts per serving: 185 cal., 3 g total fat (1 g sat. fat), 66 mg chol., 201 mg sodium, 12 g carbo., 1 g fiber, 27 g pro.
Exchanges: ½ Fruit, 4 Very Lean Meat, ½ Fat

Grilling directions: For a charcoal grill, place chicken on the lightly greased rack of an uncovered grill directly over medium coals. Grill for 12 to 15 minutes or until chicken is tender and no longer pink (170°F). (For a gas grill, preheat grill. Reduce heat to medium. Place chicken on lightly greased grill rack over heat. Cover and grill as above.)

*See note, page 76

For Wave 1, this is not appropriate. For Waves 2 and 3, serve with steamed green beans and cooked bulgur.

Wine Pairing: sparkling semisweet

SAUTÉED CHICKEN BREASTS WITH BABY GREENS AND ROASTED PEPPER SAUCE

Thinly sliced chicken piled on a bed of sweet and savory vegetables makes this a supreme main-dish salad. Roasted sweet peppers give this salad spunk and contribute vitamin C.

Prep: 30 minutes **Cook:** 8 minutes **Makes:** 4 servings

2 tablespoons extra-virgin olive oil

1 pound skinless, boneless chicken breast halves

1 15-ounce jar roasted red and yellow bell peppers, drained and chopped

½ cup chopped red onion

¼ cup capers, rinsed and drained

3 tablespoons red wine vinegar

2 tablespoons chopped fresh basil

1 tablespoon chopped fresh flat-leaf parsley

¼ teaspoon kosher salt

¼ teaspoon freshly ground black pepper

4 cups torn mixed greens

1. In a large skillet heat 2 teaspoons of the olive oil over medium heat. Add chicken; cook for 8 to 12 minutes or until chicken is no longer pink (170°F), turning once.

2. Meanwhile, in a medium bowl combine the remaining 4 teaspoons olive oil, the roasted peppers, red onion, capers, vinegar, basil, parsley, kosher salt, and black pepper. Stir until well mixed.

3. To serve, arrange mixed greens on a serving platter; spoon roasted pepper mixture over greens. Thinly slice chicken. Place on top of pepper mixture.

Nutrition facts per serving: 219 cal., 8 g total fat (1 g sat. fat), 66 mg chol., 445 mg sodium, 8 g carbo., 3 g fiber, 28 g pro.
Exchanges: 2 Vegetable, 3½ Very Lean Meat, 1 Fat

For Wave 1, serve with cooked barley. For Waves 2 and 3, serve with cooked barley and kiwi fruit.

Wine Pairing: Sauvignon Blanc

Olive Oil

Bell Peppers

SONOMA express PESTO CHICKEN AND SQUASH

Pesto, the quintessential Italian sauce, adds flavor and fragrance to this quick and easy recipe.

Start to Finish: 25 minutes **Makes:** 4 servings

1   tablespoon extra-virgin olive oil

1   pound skinless, boneless chicken breast halves, cut into thin bite-size strips

2   cups chopped yellow summer squash and/or zucchini

2   tablespoons refrigerated basil pesto

3   cups fresh spinach

1   cup cherry tomatoes, halved

    Kosher salt

    Freshly ground black pepper

2   cups hot cooked multigrain pasta (such as Barilla Plus)

2   tablespoons finely shredded Asiago or Parmesan cheese

1. In a large skillet heat olive oil over medium-high heat. Add chicken strips and squash; cook and stir for 4 to 6 minutes or until chicken is no longer pink. Stir in pesto. Add spinach and tomatoes; cook and toss about 1 minute or just until spinach is wilted. Season to taste with kosher salt and pepper. Serve over hot cooked pasta and sprinkle with cheese.

Nutrition facts per serving: 347 cal., 12 g total fat (2 g sat. fat), 71 mg chol., 310 mg sodium, 25 g carbo., 4 g fiber, 35 g pro.
Exchanges: 1½ Vegetable, 1 Starch, 4 Very Lean Meat, 2 Fat

For Wave 1, serve as is. For Waves 2 and 3, serve with fresh peach slices.

Wine Pairing: Sauvignon Blanc

Olive Oil

Tomatoes

Spinach

Whole Grains

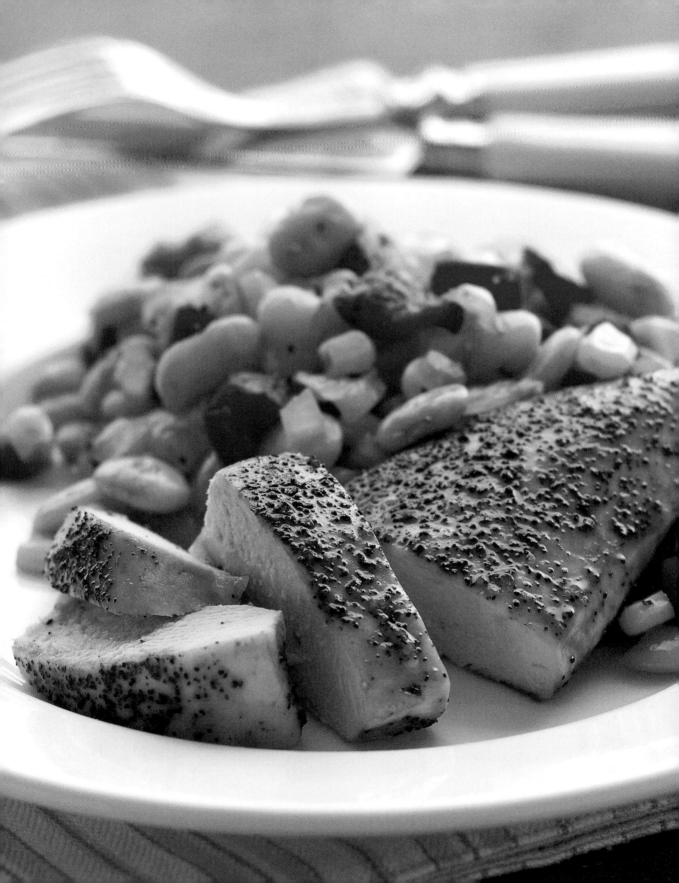

SAUTÉED CHICKEN WITH BALSAMIC SUCCOTASH

Succotash, a favorite among Southerners in the United States, sets the stage for slightly spicy chicken breasts. You'll find most of the micronutrients for this dish in the succotash. Lima beans have B vitamins, red bell pepper offers vitamin C, and they both contribute fiber.

Start to Finish: 35 minutes **Makes:** 4 servings

2 teaspoons chili powder

¼ teaspoon kosher salt

4 skinless, boneless chicken breast halves (1 to 1¼ pounds total)

2 tablespoons extra-virgin olive oil

4 cloves garlic, minced (2 teaspoons minced)

1 cup chopped sweet onion (such as Vidalia, Walla Walla, or Maui)

1 cup chopped red bell pepper

2 cups loose-pack frozen lima beans

1½ cups fresh or frozen corn kernels

2 tablespoons balsamic vinegar

Kosher salt

Freshly ground black pepper

Olive Oil

Bell Peppers

1. In a small bowl combine chili powder and the ¼ teaspoon kosher salt. Sprinkle evenly over chicken breast halves. In a large skillet heat 1 tablespoon of the olive oil over medium heat. Add chicken; cook for 10 to 12 minutes or until chicken is tender and no longer pink (170°F), turning once. Remove chicken from skillet; cover and keep warm.

2. Add the remaining 1 tablespoon olive oil to the skillet. Add garlic. Cook over low heat for 4 minutes, stirring occasionally. Increase heat to medium; add onion and bell pepper. Cook about 5 minutes or until tender, stirring occasionally. Add lima beans, corn, and balsamic vinegar; cook for 5 minutes, stirring occasionally. Season to taste with additional kosher salt and black pepper.

3. Serve chicken with lima bean mixture.

Nutrition facts per serving: 369 cal., 9 g total fat (1 g sat. fat), 66 mg chol., 380 mg sodium, 39 g carbo., 8 g fiber, 34 g pro.
Exchanges: ½ Vegetable, 2 Starch, 4 Very Lean Meat, 1½ Fat

For Wave 1, this is not appropriate. For Waves 2 and 3, serve with fresh strawberries.

Wine Pairing: Chardonnay

CILANTRO CHICKEN WITH PEANUTS

This skillet dish sizzles with flavors of Asian cuisine. A bed of shredded cabbage rounds out the dish and offers a healthful dose of vitamin A, folic acid, and potassium.

Start to Finish: 25 minutes **Makes:** 4 servings

2 teaspoons toasted canola oil

1 pound skinless, boneless chicken breast halves, cut into 1-inch strips

1 ounce honey-roasted peanuts

2 teaspoons minced fresh ginger

4 cloves garlic, minced (2 teaspoons minced)

¼ cup sliced green onions

1 tablespoon soy sauce

2 teaspoons rice vinegar

1 teaspoon toasted sesame oil

1 cup fresh cilantro leaves

4 cups finely shredded Chinese (napa) cabbage or 2 cups hot cooked brown rice

Fresh cilantro sprigs (optional)

Lime wedges (optional)

1. In a heavy 10-inch skillet heat canola oil over high heat. Add chicken; cook and stir for 2 minutes. Add peanuts, ginger, and garlic; cook and stir about 3 minutes more or until chicken is no longer pink.

2. Add green onions, soy sauce, rice vinegar, and sesame oil. Cook and stir for 2 minutes more. Remove from heat. Stir in cilantro leaves.

3. To serve, spoon chicken mixture over cabbage or rice. If desired, garnish with cilantro sprigs and lime wedges.

Nutrition facts per serving: 222 cal., 9 g total fat (2 g sat. fat), 66 mg chol., 362 mg sodium, 7 g carbo., 2 g fiber, 30 g pro.
Exchanges: 1½ Vegetable, 4 Very Lean Meat, 1 Fat

For Wave 1, serve wtih cooked brown rice and cooked bell peppers. For Waves 2 and 3, serve with cooked brown rice and fresh plum wedges.

Wine Pairing: Chardonnay

FETA-STUFFED CHICKEN

Unlike most recipes for stuffed chicken, this one requires no pounding.
Stuffed with tangy feta and served over a wilted spinach salad with toasted nuts,
this stuffed chicken recipe has all the flavor with half the work.

Start to Finish: 30 minutes **Makes:** 4 servings

1 ounce basil-and-tomato feta cheese
(¼ cup)*

2 tablespoons light tub-style cream cheese
(1 ounce)

1 tablespoon chopped fresh mint

4 skinless, boneless chicken breast halves
(1¼ to 1½ pounds total)

¼ teaspoon freshly ground black pepper

Dash kosher salt

1 tablespoon extra-virgin olive oil

¼ cup chicken broth

1 10-ounce package prewashed
fresh spinach

2 tablespoons walnut or pecan
pieces, toasted

1 tablespoon lemon juice

Lemon slices, halved (optional)

Olive Oil

Spinach

1. In a small bowl combine feta cheese, cream cheese, and mint; set aside. Using a sharp knife, cut a 1½-inch horizontal slit through the thickest portion of each chicken breast half to form a pocket that is about 1 inch deep. Stuff pockets with the cheese mixture. Secure openings with wooden toothpicks. Season chicken with pepper and kosher salt.

2. In a large nonstick skillet heat oil over medium-high heat. Add chicken; cook for 12 to 15 minutes or until tender and no longer pink (170°F.), turning occasionally to brown evenly (reduce heat to medium if chicken browns too quickly). Remove chicken from skillet. Cover and keep warm.

3. Remove skillet from heat for 1 minute. Carefully add chicken broth to skillet. Return to heat; bring to boiling. Gradually add spinach to skillet, cooking and tossing with tongs just until spinach is wilted (should take 2 to 3 minutes total). Stir in the nuts and lemon juice.

4. To serve, divide spinach mixture among four dinner plates. Top with chicken breasts. If desired, garnish with lemon slices.

Nutrition facts per serving: 266 cal., 11 g total fat (3 g sat. fat), 92 mg chol., 345 mg sodium, 4 g carbo., 2 g fiber, 37 g pro.
Exchanges: 1 Vegetable, 5 Very Lean Meat, 1½ Fat

*Note: If you can't find basil-and-tomato feta cheese, stir 1 teaspoon finely chopped fresh basil and 1 teaspoon snipped oil-packed dried tomatoes, drained, into 1 ounce (¼ cup crumbled) plain feta cheese.

For Wave 1, serve with cooked quinoa and cooked zucchini. For Waves 2 and 3, serve with cooked quinoa and fresh berries.

Wine Pairing: Sauvignon Blanc

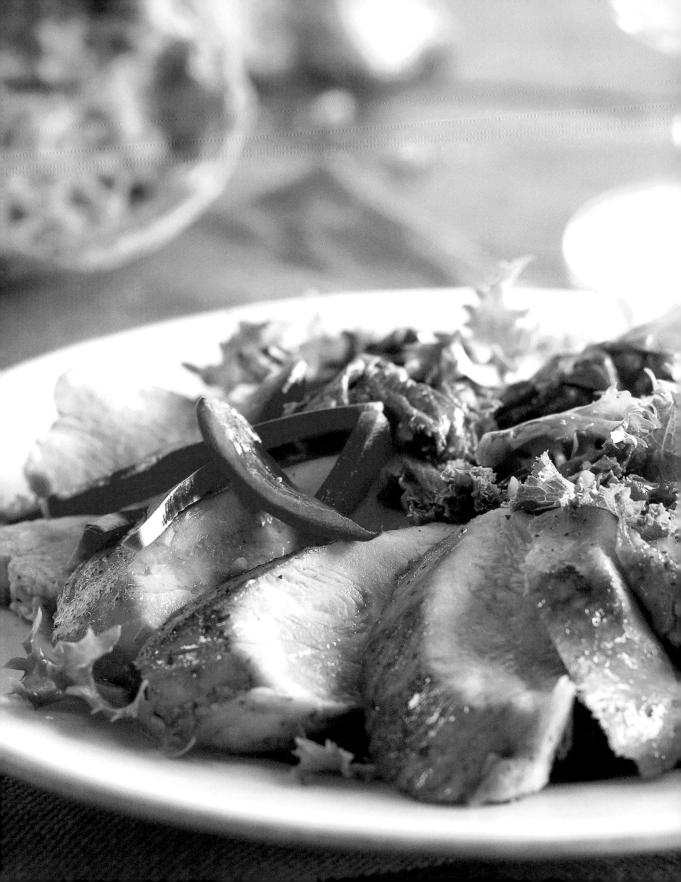

DOWN-HOME CHICKEN AND GREENS

A pound of greens may sound like a lot, but they will cook down to a more manageable amount. Remember when choosing your greens that darker greens are more nutritious. Using any of the listed options will ensure you get a big dose of vitamin C.

Start to Finish: 40 minutes **Makes:** 4 servings

4   skinless, boneless chicken breast halves (1 to 1¼ pounds total)

¼   teaspoon freshly ground black pepper

⅛   teaspoon kosher salt

     Nonstick olive oil cooking spray

⅔   cup reduced-sodium chicken broth

6   to 8 cloves garlic, minced (3 to 4 teaspoons minced)

¼   teaspoon crushed red pepper

¼   teaspoon freshly ground black pepper

1   pound fresh greens (such as mustard, Swiss chard, chicory, beet, kohlrabi, kale, collard, and/or turnip greens), torn

     Balsamic vinegar

     Red bell pepper slices (optional)

Olive Oil

Bell Peppers

1. Season chicken with ¼ teaspoon black pepper and the kosher salt. Coat an unheated very large skillet with nonstick cooking spray. Preheat over medium heat. Add chicken; cook until browned, turning to brown evenly. Reduce heat to medium-low. Cover and cook for 10 to 12 minutes or until chicken is tender and no longer pink (170°F). Remove chicken from skillet. Cover to keep warm.

2. Add broth, garlic, crushed red pepper, and ¼ teaspoon black pepper to the same skillet. Bring to boiling. Stir in greens; reduce heat. Cook for 4 to 6 minutes or just until greens are tender, stirring occasionally.

3. Spoon greens and their juices onto four dinner plates. If desired, slice chicken. Place chicken on top of greens. Drizzle lightly with balsamic vinegar. If desired, garnish with bell pepper slices.

Nutrition facts per serving: 161 cal., 2 g total fat (0 g sat. fat), 66 mg chol., 351 mg sodium, 7 g carbo., 3 g fiber, 30 g pro.
Exchanges: 1½ Vegetable, 4 Very Lean Meat

For Wave 1, serve with cooked quinoa. For Waves 2 and 3, serve with cooked quinoa and fresh apple slices.

Wine Pairing: Pinot Grigio

SONOMA *express* CHICKEN WITH HERB RUB

Cultivated throughout the Mediterranean, fennel enhances the flavor and aroma of this simple chicken dish. The flavor of fennel is similar to anise (licoricelike) but sweeter and less pungent. Experiment with the range given to determine what level of fennel is most pleasing to your palate.

Start to Finish: 25 minutes **Makes:** 4 servings

4   skinless, boneless chicken breast halves
    (1 to 1¼ pounds total)

½   cup chopped fresh mint

2   tablespoons sesame seeds

2   to 4 teaspoons fennel seeds, crushed

2   teaspoons dried thyme, crushed

1   teaspoon kosher salt

¼   teaspoon freshly ground black pepper

1   tablespoon extra-virgin olive oil

Olive Oil

1. Place a chicken breast half between 2 pieces of plastic wrap. Using the flat side of a meat mallet, pound chicken lightly to ½-inch thickness. Remove plastic wrap. Repeat with remaining chicken breast halves.

2. In a small bowl combine mint, sesame seeds, fennel seeds, thyme, kosher salt, and pepper. Sprinkle mint mixture evenly over chicken; rub in with your fingers.

3. In a very large skillet heat olive oil over medium heat. Add chicken; cook for 8 to 10 minutes or until no longer pink.

Nutrition facts per serving: 194 cal., 7 g total fat (1 g sat. fat), 66 mg chol., 543 mg sodium, 2 g carbo., 1 g fiber, 27 g pro.
Exchanges: 4 Very Lean Meat, 1 Fat

For Wave 1, serve with Basil Quinoa with Red Bell Pepper (page 221) and Tomatoes with Crispy Bread Topping (page 207). For Waves 2 and 3, serve with Basil Quinoa with Red Bell Pepper (page 221), Tomatoes with Crispy Bread Topping (page 207), and fresh grapefruit.

Wine Pairing: Pinot Grigio

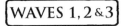

CHICKEN BREASTS WITH MEXICAN-STYLE RUB

Broiled chicken breasts offer a fuss-free weeknight dinner. The only work involved is assembling the flavorful rub that gives this dish a memorable taste of Mexico.

Prep: 15 minutes **Broil:** 12 minutes **Makes:** 4 servings

1   tablespoon dried oregano

1   tablespoon dried thyme

1   teaspoon coriander seeds

1   teaspoon anise seeds

¼   cup chili powder

1   teaspoon paprika

½   teaspoon cracked black pepper

¼   teaspoon kosher salt

4   skinless, boneless chicken breast halves
    (1 to 1¼ pounds total)

1. Preheat broiler. For rub, using a mortar and pestle, grind together the oregano, thyme, coriander seeds, and anise seeds. Stir in chili powder, paprika, pepper, and kosher salt. Sprinkle 2 teaspoons of the rub° evenly over chicken; rub in with your fingers.

2. Place chicken on the unheated rack of a broiler pan. Broil 4 to 5 inches from heat for 12 to 15 minutes or until chicken is tender and no longer pink (170°F), turning once halfway through broiling.

Nutrition facts per serving: 128 cal., 1 g total fat (0 g sat. fat), 66 mg chol., 78 mg sodium, 1 g carbo., 0 g fiber, 26 g pro.
Exchanges: 4 Very Lean Meat

Grilling directions: For a charcoal grill, place chicken on the rack of an uncovered grill directly over medium coals. Grill for 12 to 15 minutes or until chicken is tender and no longer pink (170°F), turning once halfway through grilling. (For a gas grill, preheat grill. Reduce heat to medium. Place chicken on grill rack over heat. Cover and grill as above.)

*Note: Place remaining rub in an airtight container; store at room temperature and use within 3 months.

For Wave 1, serve with cooked quinoa and steamed broccoli with bell peppers. For Waves 2 and 3, serve with Spicy Black-Eyed Pea Salad (page 216) and fresh papaya.

Wine Pairing: rosé

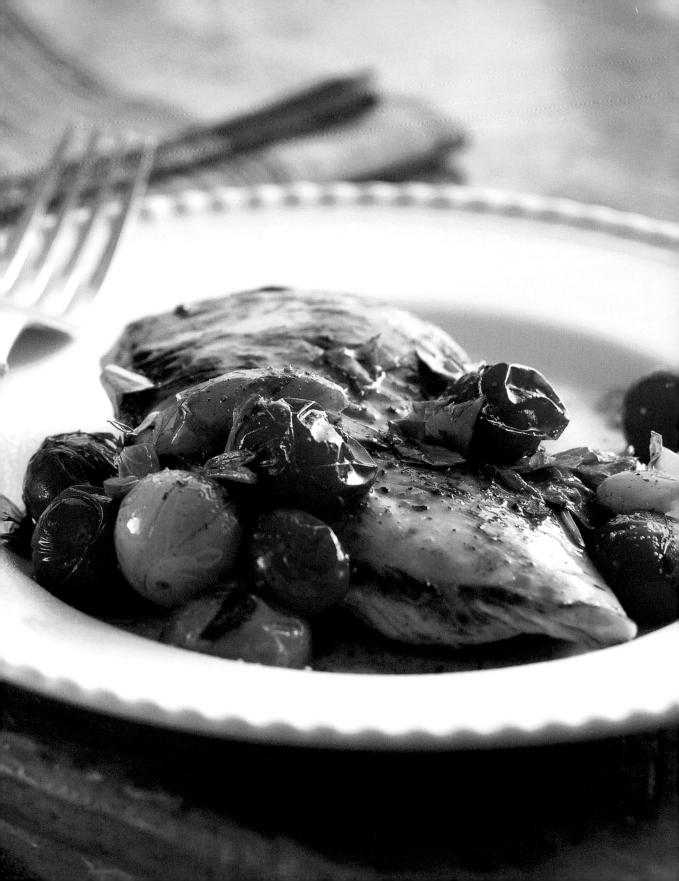

CHICKEN WITH RED AND YELLOW CHERRY TOMATOES

A simple topping of delightfully tangy red and yellow cherry tomatoes makes this meal perfect weeknight fare. Cooking the tomatoes boosts their antioxidant availability and gives them a richer flavor.

Prep: 15 minutes **Cook:** 10 minutes **Makes:** 4 servings

4 skinless, boneless chicken breast halves (1 to 1¼ pounds total)

½ teaspoon kosher salt

¼ teaspoon freshly ground black pepper

1 tablespoon extra-virgin olive oil

4 cups red and/or yellow cherry tomatoes, halved

2 tablespoons water

¼ cup chopped fresh flat-leaf parsley or basil or 2 tablespoon chopped fresh tarragon

2 tablespoons white wine vinegar

Olive Oil

Tomatoes

1. Sprinkle chicken with ¼ teaspoon of the kosher salt and ⅛ teaspoon of the pepper. In a large nonstick skillet heat olive oil over medium-high heat. Add chicken; cook for 10 to 12 minutes or until chicken is no longer pink (170°F), turning once. Transfer chicken to a serving platter; cover and keep warm.

2. Drain fat from skillet. Add tomatoes, the water, parsley, vinegar, the remaining ¼ teaspoon salt, and the remaining ⅛ teaspoon pepper to skillet. Bring to boiling; reduce heat. Simmer, uncovered, for 3 to 4 minutes or until tomatoes begin to soften, stirring occasionally. Serve the tomato mixture over chicken.

Nutrition facts per serving: 191 cal., 5 g total fat (1 g sat. fat), 66 mg chol., 327 mg sodium, 7 g carbo., 2 g fiber, 28 g pro.
Exchanges: 1 Vegetable, 4 Very Lean Meat, ½ Fat

For Wave 1, serve with cooked multigrain pasta and Roasted Green Beans with Red Onion and Walnuts (page 212). For Waves 2 and 3, serve with cooked multigrain pasta and fresh banana slices.

Wine Pairing: White Zinfandel or Pinot Noir

BISTRO CHICKEN AND GARLIC

Garlic is a powerful herb with a celebrated culinary and medicinal history. Egyptians were fed garlic for strength, and medieval healers suggested its use to ward off vampires. Today it's commended for its cancer-fighting antioxidant, allicin. In this recipe, garlic is roasted to mellow and sweeten its flavor.

Prep: 30 minutes **Bake:** 12 minutes **Oven:** 400°F **Makes:** 4 servings

1   bulb garlic

1   tablespoon extra-virgin olive oil

4   skinless, boneless chicken breast halves (1 to 1¼ pounds total)

¼   teaspoon dried basil, crushed

¼   teaspoon dried thyme, crushed

¼   teaspoon dried rosemary, crushed

¼   teaspoon kosher salt

⅛   teaspoon freshly ground black pepper

¼   cup dry vermouth or dry white wine

Olive Oil

1. Preheat oven to 400°F. Separate cloves of garlic, discarding small papery cloves in center. Trim off stem end of each garlic clove but do not peel. (This will facilitate squeezing garlic from peel after it is cooked.)

2. In a large ovenproof skillet heat olive oil over medium-high heat. Add garlic cloves and chicken. Cook about 4 minutes or until chicken is lightly browned, turning chicken and stirring garlic cloves once. Sprinkle chicken with basil, thyme, rosemary, kosher salt, and pepper; transfer skillet to the oven. Bake, covered, for 12 to 15 minute or until chicken is tender and no longer pink (170°F) and garlic is tender.

3. Using a slotted spatula, transfer chicken to a serving platter, reserving juices in skillet; cover and keep warm. Transfer garlic cloves to a small bowl; set aside for 1 to 2 minutes to cool slightly.

4. Add vermouth or white wine to skillet. Squeeze softened garlic from skins into skillet; discard skins. On rangetop, bring garlic mixture to boiling over medium heat; reduce heat. Boil gently, uncovered, about 6 minutes or until sauce thickens slightly, stirring frequently. Pour garlic sauce over chicken. If desired, garnish with herb sprigs.

Nutrition facts per serving: 185 cal., 5 g total fat (1 g sat. fat), 66 mg chol., 197 mg sodium, 3 g carbo., 0 g fiber, 27 g pro.
Exchanges: 4 Very Lean Meat, 1 Fat

For Wave 1, serve with cooked multigrain pasta, steamed asparagus, and Tomatoes with Crispy Bread Topping (page 207). For Waves 2 and 3, serve with cooked multigrain pasta, Tomatoes with Crispy Bread Topping (page 207), and fresh berries.

Wine Pairing: Syrah or Merlot

CHICKEN WITH CARAMELIZED ONION AND TOMATO SAUCE

This dish is quick to make and especially great for summer, when tomatoes, sweet peppers, and zucchini are most bountiful.

Start to Finish: 35 minutes **Makes:** 4 servings

4 skinless, boneless chicken breast halves (1 to 1½ pounds total)

Kosher salt

Freshly ground black pepper

2 tablespoons extra-virgin olive oil

1 medium yellow, red, or green bell pepper, seeded and thinly sliced

1 small red onion, thinly sliced (about 1 cup)

6 roma tomatoes, seeded and coarsely chopped (3 cups)

½ of a small zucchini, cut into bite-size strips (½ cup)

4 cloves garlic, minced (2 teaspoons minced)

2 tablespoons balsamic vinegar

2 teaspoons chopped fresh thyme

¼ cup crumbled feta cheese (1 ounce)

1. Preheat broiler. Season chicken with kosher salt and pepper. Place chicken on the unheated rack of a broiler pan. Broil 4 to 5 inches from the heat for 12 to 15 minutes or until chicken is no longer pink (170°F), turning once halfway through broiling.

2. Meanwhile, in a large skillet heat oil over medium heat. Add bell pepper and red onion. Reduce heat to medium-low. Cook for 10 to 15 minutes or until very tender, stirring occasionally. Increase heat to medium. Add tomatoes, zucchini, and garlic; cook and stir for 2 minutes more. Stir in balsamic vinegar and thyme.

3. Thinly slice chicken. Serve chicken with tomato mixture; sprinkle with cheese.

Nutrition facts per serving: 270 cal., 10 g total fat (3 g sat. fat), 74 mg chol., 415 mg sodium, 14 g carbo., 3 g fiber, 30 g pro.
Exchanges: 2 Vegetable, 4 Very Lean Meat, 2 Fat

For Wave 1, serve with a mixed green salad and cooked multigrain pasta. For Waves 2 and 3, serve with cooked multigrain pasta and fresh banana slices.

Wine Pairing: Sauvignon Blanc

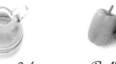

Olive Oil

Bell Peppers

Tomatoes

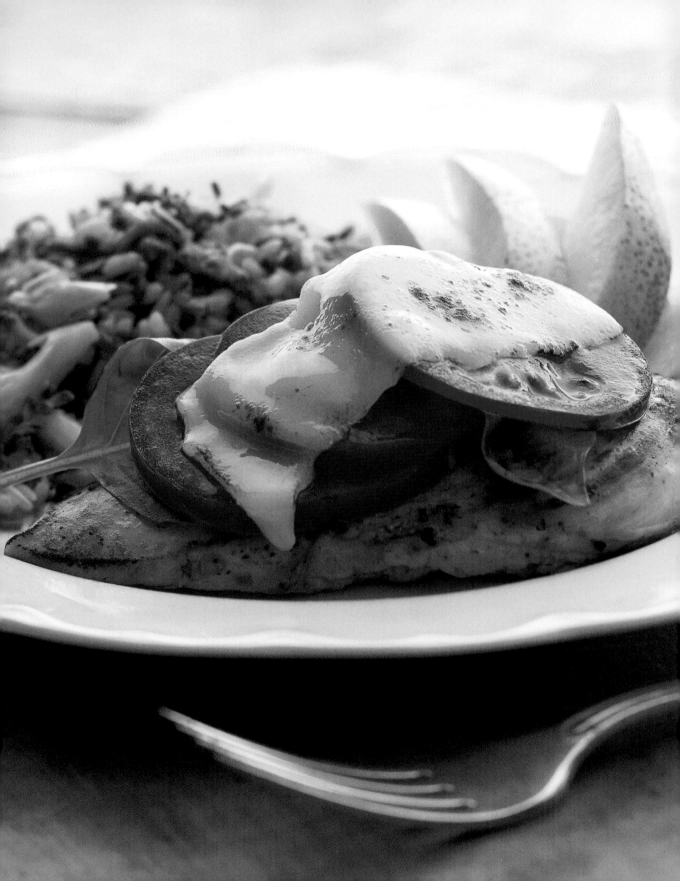

MARINATED CHICKEN BREASTS WITH MOZZARELLA

*This stunning chicken dish exudes elegance. Known to ancient Greeks as the royal herb,
basil offers intense flavor and gorgeous color as one layer of this multilayered meal.*

Prep: 25 minutes **Marinate:** 2 to 6 hours **Cook:** 45 minutes + 10 minutes **Broil:** 1 minute **Makes:** 4 servings

---

4   skinless, boneless chicken breast halves
     (1 to 1½ pounds total)

     Kosher salt

     Freshly ground black pepper

¼   cup bottled clear Italian salad dressing
     (such as Newman's Own brand)

⅓   cup wild rice

1⅓   cups reduced-sodium chicken broth

⅓   cup long grain brown rice

1   cup broccoli florets, coarsely chopped

¼   cup thinly sliced green onions

2   teaspoons extra-virgin olive oil

8   to 10 large fresh basil leaves

1   large tomato, thinly sliced

2   slices part-skim mozzarella cheese, halved
     (3 ounces)

Olive Oil

Tomatoes

Broccoli

Whole Grains

1. Season chicken with kosher salt and pepper. Place chicken in a large self-sealing plastic bag set in a shallow bowl. Pour salad dressing over chicken. Seal bag; turn to coat chicken. Marinate in the refrigerator for 2 to 6 hours, turning bag occasionally.

2 Rinse wild rice well; set aside. In a medium saucepan bring chicken broth to boiling. Add uncooked wild rice and brown rice. Return to boiling; reduce heat. Cover and simmer for 40 minutes. Quickly stir broccoli and green onions into rice mixture. Cover and simmer about 5 minutes more or until rice is tender and most of the liquid is absorbed.

3. Meanwhile, drain chicken, discarding marinade. In a large cast-iron skillet or other large broilerproof skillet heat olive oil over medium heat. Add chicken; cook for 10 to 12 minutes or until no longer pink (170°F), turning once halfway through cooking.

4. Preheat broiler. Lay basil leaves on chicken breast halves in skillet. Arrange tomato slices over basil leaves, overlapping as necessary. Top each chicken breast half with a half-slice of cheese. Broil 3 to 4 inches from heat about 1 minute or until cheese is melted and bubbly. Serve with hot rice mixture.

Nutrition facts per serving: 407 cal., 16 g total fat
(4 g sat. fat), 79 mg chol., 999 mg sodium, 29 g carbo.,
3 g fiber, 37 g pro.
Exchanges: 1 Vegetable, 1½ Starch, 4½ Very Lean Meat,
2½ Fat

---

*For Wave 1, serve as is. For Waves 2 and 3,
serve with fresh pear slices.*

Wine Pairing: *Merlot*

GARLIC AND MINT CHICKEN BREASTS

*An intriguing mint marinade bathes tender chicken breasts in cool and hot flavors simultaneously.
Fresh mint is most plentiful during summer months when you're apt to enjoy
a refreshing grilled dish like this.*

Prep: 15 minutes **Marinate:** 4 to 24 hours **Grill:** 12 minutes **Makes:** 4 servings

½ cup fresh mint leaves

1 tablespoon lemon juice

1 tablespoon extra-virgin olive oil

1 tablespoon reduced-sodium soy sauce

1 teaspoon chili powder

¼ teaspoon freshly ground black pepper

4 cloves garlic, peeled

4 skinless, boneless chicken breast halves
   (1 to 1¼ pounds total)

   Hot cooked couscous (optional)

   Fresh mint sprigs (optional)

Olive Oil

1. In a blender combine the mint leaves, lemon juice, olive oil, soy sauce, chili powder, pepper, and garlic. Cover and blend until smooth.

2. Place chicken in a self-sealing plastic bag set in a shallow dish. Pour mint mixture over chicken. Seal bag; turn to coat chicken. Marinate chicken in the refrigerator for 4 to 24 hours, turning bag occasionally.

3. For a charcoal grill, place chicken on the rack of an uncovered grill directly over medium coals. Grill for 12 to 15 minutes or until tender and no longer pink (170°F), turning once halfway through grilling. (For a gas grill, preheat grill. Reduce heat to medium. Place chicken on grill rack over heat. Cover and grill as above.)

4. If desired, serve over hot cooked couscous. If desired, garnish with mint sprigs.

Nutrition facts per serving: 202 cal., 6 g total fat (1 g sat. fat), 82 mg chol., 228 mg sodium, 2 g carbo., 0 g fiber, 34 g pro.
Exchanges: 4½ Lean Meat

For Wave 1, serve with Broccoli with Goat Cheese and Walnuts (page 211) and fresh cucumber slices. For Waves 2 and 3, serve with Broccoli with Goat Cheese and Walnuts (page 211) and fresh pear slices.

Wine Pairing: Sauvignon Blanc

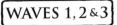

TURKEY PAILLARDS WITH ASPARAGUS AND TOMATOES

If you haven't started incorporating more soy into your diet, the sweet, delicate flavor of edamame in this yummy dish is sure to hook you. Soybeans, such as edamame, are a powerhouse of nutrients; they contain protein, fiber, phytochemicals, essential fatty acids, thiamin, and riboflavin, to name just a few.

Start to Finish: 30 minutes **Makes:** 4 servings

1 12-ounce turkey breast tenderloin

½ teaspoon kosher salt

½ teaspoon freshly ground black pepper

2 tablespoons extra-virgin olive oil

1 medium onion, sliced

1¼ pounds fresh asparagus, trimmed and bias-cut into 1-inch pieces (3 cups)

1 cup fresh or frozen shelled sweet soybeans (edamame)

¼ cup water

1 cup cherry tomatoes, halved

1 tablespoon chopped fresh basil

1 tablespoon chopped fresh thyme

2 teaspoons lemon juice

2 tablespoons pine nuts, toasted

Olive Oil

Tomatoes

1. Cut the turkey tenderloin in half horizontally. Place each half between 2 pieces of plastic wrap; gently pound with the flat side of a meat mallet to ¼-inch thickness. Cut each turkey piece in half crosswise to make 4 pieces total. Season turkey with ¼ teaspoon of the kosher salt and ¼ teaspoon of the pepper.

2. In a large skillet heat 1 tablespoon of the olive oil over medium-high heat. Add turkey to skillet in a single layer. Cook for 4 to 6 minutes or until browned and no longer pink, turning once. Transfer turkey to a serving platter; cover and keep warm.

3. In the same skillet heat the remaining 1 tablespoon olive oil over medium-high heat. Add onion; cook and stir for 2 minutes. Add asparagus, soybeans, and the water to skillet. Bring to boiling; reduce heat. Cover and cook for 3 minutes. Add cherry tomatoes, basil, thyme, lemon juice, the remaining ¼ teaspoon kosher salt, and the remaining ¼ teaspoon pepper. Stir in the pine nuts.

4. Serve asparagus mixture with the turkey.

Nutrition facts per serving: 325 cal., 15 g total fat (2 g sat. fat), 53 mg chol., 289 mg sodium, 18 g carbo., 7 g fiber, 34 g pro.
Exchanges: 1½ Vegetable, ½ Starch, 4 Very Lean Meat, 2½ Fat

For Wave 1, serve with Wine Country Grain Medley (page 220). For Waves 2 and 3, serve with Brown Rice Pilaf (page 217) and fresh peach slices.

Wine Pairing: Sauvignon Blanc

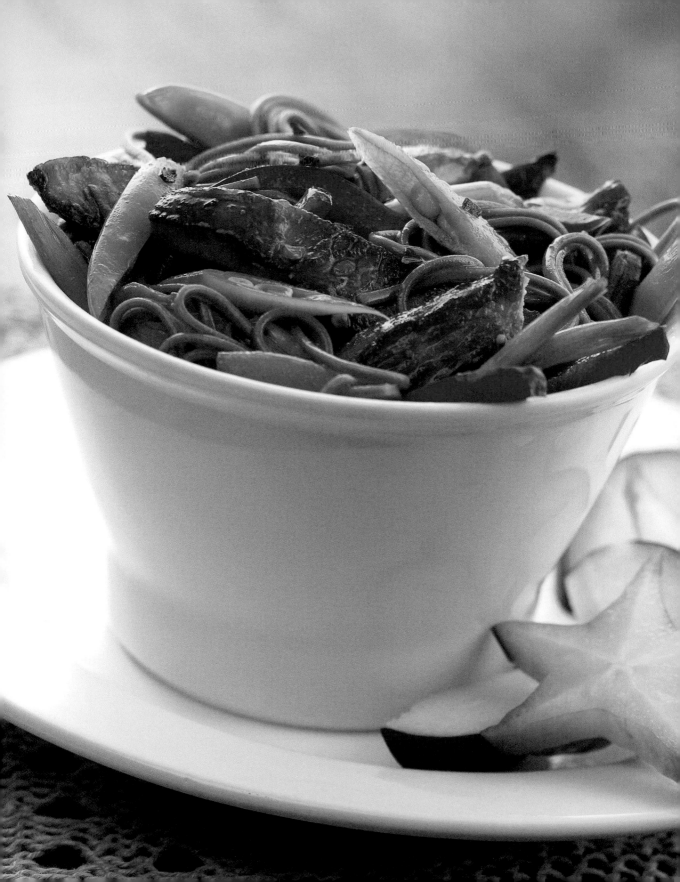

TURKEY AND SOBA NOODLE STIR-FRY

Japanese buckwheat noodles are amazingly versatile and becoming increasingly popular among Western cooks as their nutty flavor and nutritional value are realized. As the foundation of this vitamin C-rich stir-fry, buckwheat noodles add additional protein and fiber.

Start to Finish: 25 minutes **Makes:** 4 servings

6	ounces dried soba (buckwheat) noodles or multigrain spaghetti
2	teaspoons extra-virgin olive oil
2	cups fresh sugar snap peas
2	medium red bell peppers, cut into thin strips
2	teaspoons minced fresh ginger
4	cloves garlic, minced (2 teaspoons minced)
4	green onions, bias-sliced into 1-inch pieces
12	ounces turkey breast tenderloin, cut into bite-size strips
1	teaspoon toasted sesame oil
½	cup bottled plum sauce
¼	teaspoon crushed red pepper

1. Cook soba noodles according to package directions; drain. Return to hot saucepan; cover and keep warm.

2. Meanwhile, pour olive oil into a wok or large skillet. (Add more oil as necessary during cooking.) Heat over medium-high heat. Stir-fry sugar snap peas, bell peppers, ginger, and garlic in hot oil for 2 minutes. Add green onions. Stir-fry for 1 to 2 minutes more or until vegetables are crisp-tender. Remove vegetables from wok.

3. Add turkey and sesame oil to the hot wok. Stir-fry for 3 to 4 minutes or until turkey is tender and no longer pink. Add plum sauce and crushed red pepper. Return cooked vegetables to wok; stir to coat all ingredients with sauce. Heat through. Serve immediately over soba noodles.

Nutrition facts per serving: 376 cal., 5 g total fat (1 g sat. fat), 53 mg chol., 410 mg sodium, 56 g carbo., 5 g fiber, 29 g pro.
Exchanges: 1½ Vegetable, 2 Starch, 1 Other Carbo., 3 Very Lean Meat, ½ Fat

For Wave 1, this is not appropriate. For Waves 2 and 3, serve with fresh starfruit and fresh apricot slices.

Wine Pairing: sparkling semisweet

Olive Oil

Bell Peppers

Whole Grains

TURKEY MEAT LOAF

Sure, the type of meat is changed, but this meat loaf has plenty of classic flavor and homey feeling. Topped with a sweet, saucy glaze of honey, tomato sauce, and cumin, this dish could easily become your new favorite comfort food.

Prep: 25 minutes **Bake:** 45 minutes + 15 minutes **Stand:** 10 minutes **Oven:** 350°F **Makes:** 8 to 10 servings

2 teaspoons extra-virgin olive oil
¾ cup finely chopped onion
½ cup finely chopped celery
½ cup finely chopped green bell pepper
3 cloves garlic, minced (1½ teaspoons minced)
1½ pounds uncooked ground turkey
¾ cup quick-cooking rolled oats
¼ cup chicken broth
¼ cup tomato sauce
1 slightly beaten egg
½ teaspoon ground cumin
1 teaspoon freshly ground black pepper
¼ cup tomato sauce
1 tablespoon honey
½ teaspoon ground cumin

1. Preheat oven to 350°F. Line a 9×5×3-inch loaf pan with foil, letting foil extend slightly over sides; set aside. In a large skillet heat olive oil over medium heat. Add onion, celery, bell pepper, and garlic; cook about 5 minutes or until tender, stirring occasionally.

2. In a large bowl combine the cooked vegetables, ground turkey, oats, chicken broth, ¼ cup tomato sauce, the egg, ½ teaspoon cumin, and the black pepper. Mix well. Spoon into prepared pan; press firmly. Bake for 45 minutes.

3. Meanwhile, in a small bowl combine ¼ cup tomato sauce, the honey, and ½ teaspoon cumin. Spoon over meat loaf in pan. Bake for 15 to 25 minutes more or until juices run clear and an instant-read thermometer inserted in center of meat loaf registers 165°F.

4. Let meat loaf stand in pan on a wire rack for 10 minutes. Carefully lift meat loaf from pan using foil. Using a large spatula, transfer meat loaf from foil to a serving platter. Slice to serve.

Nutrition facts per serving: 202 cal., 9 g total fat (2 g sat. fat), 94 mg chol., 187 mg sodium, 11 g carbo., 2 g fiber, 18 g pro.
Exchanges: ½ Starch, 2½ Very Lean Meat, 1½ Fat

For Wave 1, this is not appropriate. For Waves 2 and 3, serve with a whole grain roll, a baked sweet potato, and fresh apple slices.

Wine Pairing: Merlot

Olive Oil

Bell Peppers

Whole Grains

SONOMA express GRILLED TURKEY PAILLARDS

"Paillard" is a term describing thinly sliced cuts of meat or meat lightly pounded into flattened pieces that are then sautéed or grilled quickly. This recipe uses the grilling method, but if weather is not permitting, sauté these paillards with a tablespoon of olive oil in a skillet.

Prep: 25 minutes **Grill:** 4 minutes **Makes:** 4 servings

2 tablespoons extra-virgin olive oil

1 tablespoon chopped fresh flat-leaf parsley

1 tablespoon chopped fresh thyme

1 tablespoon chopped fresh sage

4 cloves garlic, minced (2 teaspoons minced)

¼ teaspoon kosher salt

¼ teaspoon freshly ground black pepper

1 pound turkey breast tenderloins

Olive Oil

1. In a small bowl stir together the olive oil, parsley, thyme, sage, garlic, kosher salt, and pepper; set aside.

2. Cut the turkey tenderloins crosswise into 1-inch-thick slices. Place each slice, cut side up, between 2 pieces of plastic wrap. Using the flat side of a meat mallet, pound the turkey to ¼-inch thickness. Arrange turkey slices on a tray or baking sheet. Spread with the herb mixture.

3. For a charcoal grill, place the turkey, herb sides down, on the rack of an uncovered grill directly over medium coals. Grill for 4 to 6 minutes or until turkey is tender and no longer pink, turning once halfway through grilling. (For a gas grill, preheat grill. Reduce heat to medium. Place turkey, herb sides down, on the grill rack over heat. Cover and grill as above.)

Nutrition facts per serving: 194 cal., 8 g total fat (1 g sat. fat), 70 mg chol., 177 mg sodium, 2 g carbo., 1 g fiber, 28 g pro.
Exchanges: 4 Very Lean Meat, 1½ Fat

Rangetop directions: In a large skillet heat 1 tablespoon extra-virgin olive oil over medium-high heat. Cook turkey, half at a time, for 4 to 6 minutes or until turkey is no longer pink, turning once halfway through cooking.

For Wave 1, serve with cooked multigrain pasta, steamed asparagus, and Stuffed Cherry Tomatoes (page 249). For Waves 2 and 3, serve with cooked multigrain pasta, Stuffed Cherry Tomatoes (page 249), and fresh berries.

Wine Pairing: Pinot Noir or sparkling Pinot Noir

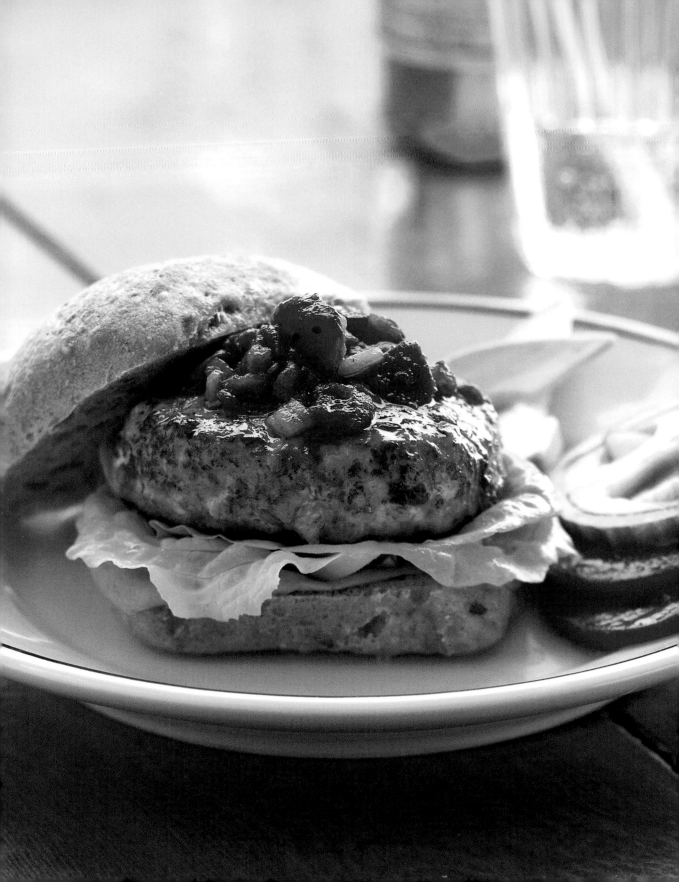

GRILLED MUSHROOM TURKEY BURGERS

Italian flat-leaf parsley is no garnish in these juicy burgers; it's a key ingredient that adds color, flavor, and vitamins A and C. Top your burger with any of the suggested condiments for a more filling meal.

Prep: 15 minutes **Stand:** 20 minutes **Grill:** 14 minutes **Makes:** 4 servings

2   tablespoons dried porcini or shiitake mushrooms

1   cup boiling water

12 ounces ground turkey breast

½   cup bottled salsa

¼   cup finely chopped onion

2   tablespoons chopped fresh flat-leaf parsley

6   cloves garlic, minced (1 tablespoon minced)

2   teaspoons chopped fresh sage

¼   teaspoon kosher salt

⅛   teaspoon freshly ground black pepper

4   whole wheat hamburger buns, split and toasted (optional)

Lettuce leaves, bottled salsa, sliced red onion, sliced avocado, and/or sliced tomato (optional)

Whole Grains

Tomatoes

1. Rinse dried mushrooms well. Place mushrooms in a small bowl; add the boiling water. Let stand about 20 minutes or until soft. Drain the mushrooms well; finely chop mushrooms.

2. In a medium bowl combine the mushrooms, turkey, the ½ cup salsa, the onion, parsley, garlic, sage, kosher salt, and pepper. Shape mixture into four ¾-inch-thick patties.

3. For a charcoal grill, place patties on the greased rack of an uncovered grill directly over medium coals. Grill for 14 to 18 minutes or until no longer pink (165°F),° turning once halfway through grilling. (For a gas grill, preheat grill. Reduce heat to medium. Place burgers on the greased grill rack over heat. Cover and grill as above.)

4. If desired, serve burgers on whole wheat buns with lettuce, additional salsa, sliced red onion, sliced avocado, and/or sliced tomato.

Nutrition facts per serving: 119 cal., 1 g total fat (0 g sat. fat), 34 mg chol., 281 mg sodium, 7 g carbo., 1 g fiber, 21 g pro.
Exchanges: ½ Vegetable, 3 Very Lean Meat

*Note: The internal color of a burger is not a reliable doneness indicator. A turkey patty cooked to 165°F is safe, regardless of color. To measure the doneness of a patty, insert an instant-read thermometer through the side of the patty to a depth of 2 to 3 inches.

For Wave 1, serve with the optional ingredients and a tossed green salad. For Waves 2 and 3, serve with the optional ingredients and fresh honeydew melon.

Wine Pairing: sparkling Pinot Noir

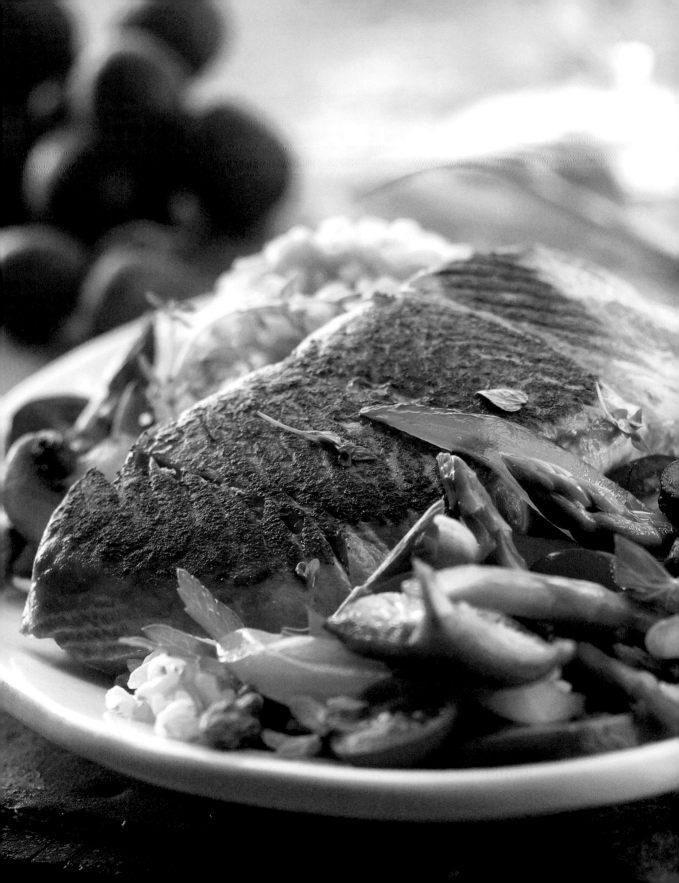

Fish & Seafood

Do you avoid fish and seafood because they are a hassle to cook? Or because you find the taste too dull or too fishy? Get ready for some recipes that will change your outlook. Braised halibut, grilled salmon, baked snapper, sautéed shrimp, and lots more are a snap to cook once you give them a try. And you'll find that the scrumptious taste of these seafood dishes is rivaled only by their heart and weight loss benefits.

BROILED HALIBUT WITH BALSAMIC GLAZE

A glaze featuring balsamic vinegar, soy sauce, honey, and garlic turns a basic halibut fillet into an extraordinary entree.

Prep: 20 minutes **Marinate:** 30 minutes to 1½ hours **Broil:** 8 minutes **Makes:** 4 servings

4   4- to 6-ounce fresh or frozen halibut fillets, about 1 inch thick

½   cup balsamic vinegar

2   tablespoons soy sauce

2   tablespoons extra-virgin olive oil

2   tablespoons honey

2   cloves garlic, minced (1 teaspoon minced)

1   teaspoon chopped fresh basil

Olive Oil

1. Thaw halibut, if frozen. Rinse fish; pat dry with paper towels. Set aside.

2. For marinade, in a shallow dish combine balsamic vinegar, soy sauce, olive oil, honey, garlic, and basil. Add halibut; turn to coat with marinade. Cover and marinate in the refrigerator for 30 minutes to 1½ hours, turning fish occasionally.

3. Preheat broiler. Drain fish, reserving marinade. Place fish on the greased unheated rack of a broiler pan. Broil 4 inches from the heat for 8 to 12 minutes or until fish flakes easily when tested with a fork, turning once halfway through broiling.

4. Meanwhile, for glaze, pour reserved marinade into a small saucepan. Bring to boiling; reduce heat. Simmer, uncovered, for 5 to 10 minutes or until thickened and reduced to ⅓ cup. Serve glaze over halibut fillets.

Nutrition facts per serving: 243 cal., 9 g total fat (1 g sat. fat), 36 mg chol., 569 mg sodium, 14 g carbo., 0 g fiber, 24 g pro.
Exchanges: 1 Other Carbo., 3½ Very Lean Meat, 1½ Fat

For Wave 1, this is not appropriate. For Waves 2 and 3, serve with a mixed green salad, cooked wild rice, and fresh apricot slices.

Wine Pairing: Sangiovese

SPICY SMOKED PEPPER HALIBUT

Delicate, mildly flavored halibut is graced with warm Mexican flavors for a smoky, piquant dish.

Prep: 15 minutes **Marinate:** 30 minutes **Grill:** 8 minutes **Makes:** 6 servings

6 4-ounce fresh or frozen halibut, swordfish, or shark steaks, cut 1 inch thick

1 medium red bell pepper, seeded and cut up

2 canned chipotle chile peppers in adobo sauce*

1 tablespoon adobo sauce from canned chipotle chile peppers in adobo sauce

2 tablespoons lime juice

2 cloves garlic, halved

1 teaspoon dried oregano

⅛ teaspoon kosher salt

¼ teaspoon kosher salt

Bell Peppers

1. Thaw fish, if frozen. Rinse fish; pat dry with paper towels. Set aside.

2. For marinade, in a blender or food processor combine bell pepper, chipotle peppers, adobo sauce, lime juice, garlic, oregano, and the ⅛ teaspoon kosher salt. Cover and blend until pureed. Reserve half of the marinade mixture to serve with fish.

3. Place fish in a shallow glass dish. Spoon remaining half of the marinade over the fish, spreading evenly. Turn fish once to coat with marinade. Cover and marinate in the refrigerator for 30 minutes.

4. Season fish with the ¼ teaspoon kosher salt. For a charcoal grill, place fish on the greased rack of an uncovered grill directly over medium coals. Grill for 8 to 12 minutes or until fish flakes easily when tested with a fork, gently turning once halfway through grilling. (For a gas grill, preheat grill. Reduce heat to medium. Place fish on greased grill rack over heat. Cover and grill as above.) Serve fish with the reserved marinade mixture.

*See note, page 76

Nutrition facts per serving: 136 cal., 3 g total fat (0 g sat. fat), 36 mg chol., 195 mg sodium, 3 g carbo., 1 g fiber, 24 g pro.
Exchanges: 3½ Very Lean Meat

For Wave 1, serve with cooked quinoa and Crumb-Topped Cauliflower (page 208). For Waves 2 and 3, serve with cooked quinoa, cooked corn, and fresh cantaloupe.

Wine Pairing: Sauvignon Blanc

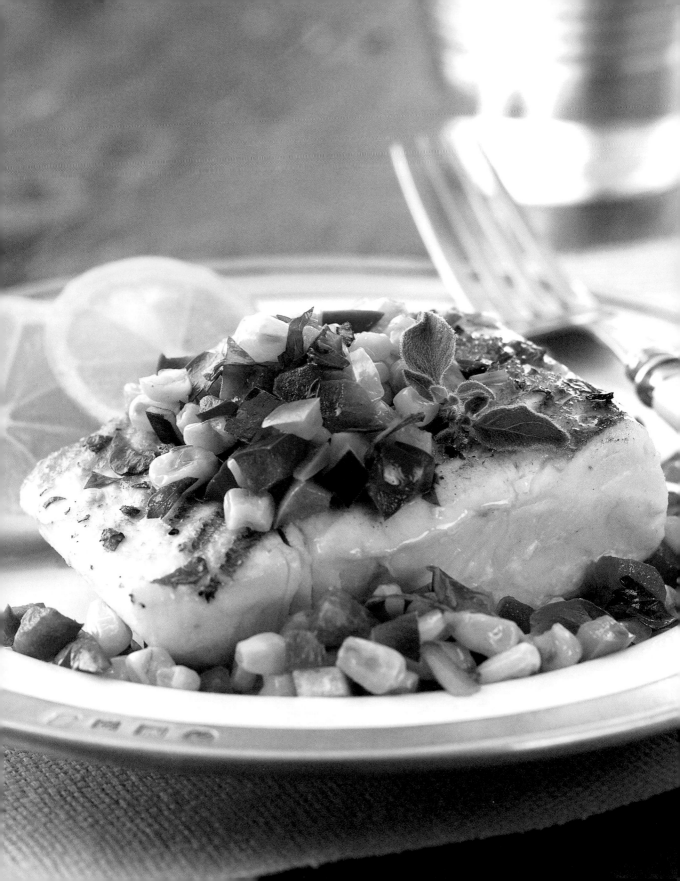

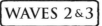
GRILLED HALIBUT WITH CORN AND PEPPER RELISH

You'll find it helpful to have your "mise en place" before starting this recipe. "Mise en place" is a French term referring to having all your ingredients measured and ready to combine.

Prep: 45 minutes **Grill:** 8 minutes **Makes:** 4 servings (plus leftover relish)

4	5- to 6-ounce fresh or frozen halibut steaks, cut 1 inch thick
	Kosher salt
	Freshly ground black pepper
3	tablespoons extra-virgin olive oil
1	tablespoon chopped fresh flat-leaf parsley
1	tablespoon chopped fresh oregano
1½	cups fresh or frozen corn kernels
1	cup finely chopped red bell pepper
1	cup finely chopped green bell pepper
2	cloves garlic, minced (1 teaspoon minced)
¼	teaspoon kosher salt
⅛	teaspoon cayenne pepper
½	cup seeded and chopped tomato
¼	cup finely chopped red onion
3	tablespoons chopped fresh flat-leaf parsley
1	tablespoon white wine vinegar
	Fresh oregano (optional)

1. Thaw fish, if frozen. Rinse fish; pat dry with paper towels. Season both sides of each halibut steak with kosher salt and black pepper. In a small bowl combine 1 tablespoon of the olive oil, the 1 tablespoon parsley, and the oregano. Rub over both sides of each halibut steak; set aside.

2. In a large skillet heat 1 tablespoon of the remaining olive oil over medium-high heat. Add corn; cook about 4 minutes or just until starting to brown, stirring occasionally. Add bell peppers; cook and stir for 2 minutes more. Stir in the garlic, the ¼ teaspoon kosher salt, and the cayenne pepper. Cook and stir for 1 minute more. Remove from the heat and let cool slightly.

3. For a charcoal grill, place fish on the rack of an uncovered grill directly over medium coals. Grill for 8 to 12 minutes or until fish flakes easily when tested with a fork, gently turning once halfway through grilling. (For a gas grill, preheat grill. Reduce heat to medium. Place fish on grill rack over heat. Cover and grill as above.)

4. Meanwhile, for relish, in a medium bowl combine corn mixture, tomato, red onion, the 3 tablespoons parsley, the white wine vinegar, and the remaining 1 tablespoon oil; toss well. Serve each halibut steak with ½ cup of the relish. Cover and chill remaining relish for another use. If desired, garnish with fresh oregano.

Nutrition facts per serving: 282 cal., 12 g total fat (2 g sat. fat), 45 mg chol., 283 mg sodium, 13 g carbo., 2 g fiber, 32 g pro.
Exchanges: ½ Vegetable, ½ Starch, 4 Very Lean Meat, 2 Fat

Broiling directions: Place fish on the unheated rack of a broiler pan. Broil 4 inches from the heat for 8 to 12 minutes or until fish flakes easily when tested with a fork, turning once halfway through broiling.

For Wave 1, this is not appropriate. For Waves 2 and 3, serve with cooked brown rice and fresh orange slices.

Wine Pairing: Chardonnay

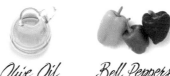

Olive Oil   *Bell Peppers*   *Tomatoes*

BROILED BBQ-SPICED RUBBED SALMON

The cooking time for this highly seasoned salmon dish depends on its thickness, but rest assured, this recipe is simple and speedy.

Start to Finish: 25 minutes **Makes:** 6 servings

6 4-ounce fresh or frozen skinless, boneless salmon fillets, about 1 inch thick

1 tablespoon sweet paprika

1 tablespoon smoked paprika or ground ancho chile pepper

1 tablespoon chili powder

1 teaspoon kosher salt

1 teaspoon garlic powder

1 teaspoon freshly ground black pepper

½ teaspoon ground cumin

½ teaspoon dried oregano, crushed

3 tablespoons extra-virgin olive oil

Olive Oil

1. Thaw fish, if frozen. Rinse fish; pat dry with paper towels. Measure thickness of fish. Set aside.

2. In a small bowl combine sweet paprika, smoked paprika, chili powder, kosher salt, garlic powder, black pepper, cumin, and oregano. Transfer spice mixture to a piece of waxed paper. Gently roll fish fillets in spice mixture to coat.

3. Brush about half of the olive oil in the bottom of a broiler pan or 15×10×1-inch baking pan. Place fish fillets in prepared pan; turn any thin portions under to make uniform thickness. Drizzle tops of fish with remaining olive oil. Broil fish 4 inches from the heat for 4 to 6 minutes per ½-inch thickness of fish or until fish flakes easily when tested with a fork, carefully turning once halfway through broiling.

Nutrition facts per serving: 280 cal., 19 g total fat (3 g sat. fat), 66 mg chol., 403 mg sodium, 3 g carbo., 2 g fiber, 23 g pro.
Exchanges: 3½ Lean Meat, 2 Fat

For Wave 1, serve with cooked barley and steamed green beans. For Waves 2 and 3, serve with cooked barley, steamed green beans, and fresh banana slices.

Wine Pairing: sparkling semisweet

GRILLED SALMON WITH HERB CRUST

Succulent salmon fillets are a good source of vitamin A, B vitamins, protein, and omega-3 fatty acids. These fillets are crusted with cilantro, oregano, and green onions for brilliant color.

Prep: 15 minutes **Grill:** 8 minutes **Makes:** 4 servings

12 ounces fresh or frozen skinless salmon fillets, about ¾ inch thick

⅓ cup coarsely chopped fresh oregano

⅓ cup coarsely chopped fresh cilantro

¼ cup sliced green onions

1 clove garlic

1 tablespoon lemon juice

2 teaspoons extra-virgin olive oil

¼ teaspoon kosher salt

⅛ teaspoon freshly ground black pepper

Olive Oil

1. Thaw salmon, if frozen. Rinse fish; pat dry with paper towels. Cut fish into two pieces (about 6 ounces). Set aside.

2. In a food processor or a mini chopper combine oregano, cilantro, green onions, garlic, lemon juice, olive oil, kosher salt, and pepper. Cover and process until chopped. (Or use a knife to finely chop the oregano, cilantro, green onions and garlic. Transfer to a shallow bowl. Stir in lemon juice, olive oil, kosher salt, and pepper.) Generously coat both sides of the salmon with the herb mixture.

3. For a charcoal grill, place salmon on the rack of an uncovered grill directly over medium-hot coals. Grill for 6 to 8 minutes or just until the salmon flakes easily when tested with a fork. (For a gas grill, preheat grill. Reduce heat to medium-high. Place salmon on grill rack over heat. Cover and grill as above.)

4. To serve, cut each salmon piece in half.

Nutrition facts per serving: 185 cal., 12 g total fat (2 g sat. fat), 50 mg chol., 176 mg sodium, 2 g carbo., 0 g fiber, 17 g pro.
Exchanges: 2½ Lean Meat, 1 Fat

For Wave 1, serve with cooked multigrain pasta and Tomatoes with Crispy Bread Topping (page 207). For Waves 2 and 3, serve with cooked multigrain pasta and Fig Salad with Fig and Port Vinaigrette (page 264).

Wine Pairing: Sauvignon Blanc

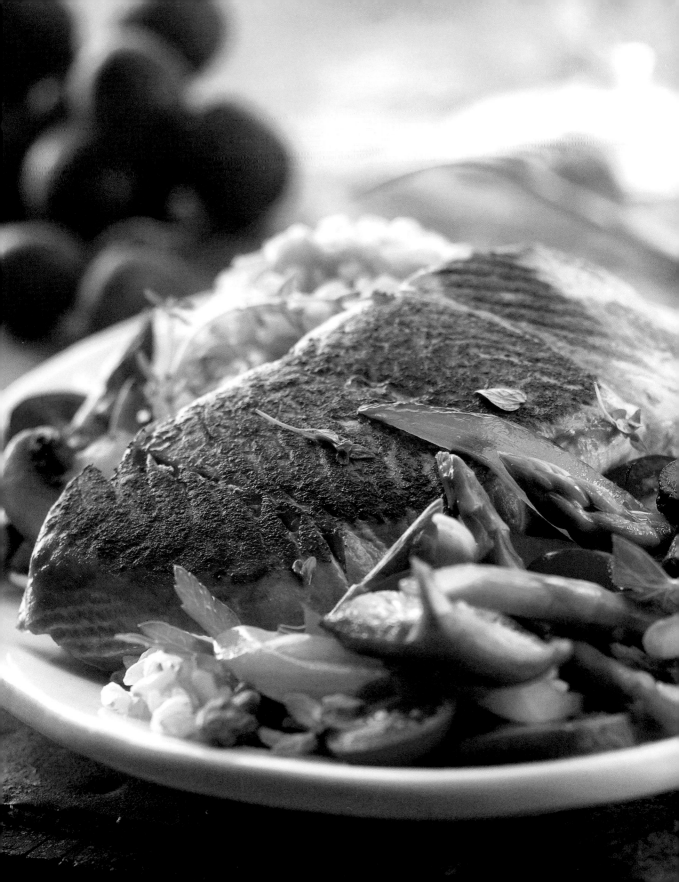

SALMON WITH ASPARAGUS AND MUSHROOMS

Very few foods naturally contain vitamin D, but you'll get a double dose with the salmon and mushrooms in this recipe.

Start to Finish: 45 minutes **Makes:** 4 servings

4 fresh or frozen skinless salmon fillets, about 1 inch thick (about 1 pound total)

Kosher salt

Freshly ground black pepper

2 tablespoons extra-virgin olive oil

2 cups sliced assorted fresh mushrooms (such as button, cremini, and/or stemmed shiitake)

1 cup chopped onion

6 cloves garlic, minced (1 tablespoon minced)

1 tablespoon chopped fresh thyme

1 cup dry white wine

1 cup clam juice, fish stock, chicken stock, or chicken broth

2 cups 1½-inch-long pieces asparagus

1 cup cherry tomatoes, halved

1 tablespoon chopped fresh flat-leaf parsley

1 teaspoon lemon juice

Fresh thyme sprigs (optional)

Olive Oil

Tomatoes

1. Thaw fish, if frozen. Rinse fish; pat dry with paper towels. Measure thickness of fish fillets. Season fish with kosher salt and pepper. Set aside.

2. In a large skillet heat 1 tablespoon of the olive oil over medium heat. Add mushrooms; cook about 5 minutes or until golden brown. Add onion, garlic, and thyme; cook until mushrooms are tender, stirring occasionally. Add wine. Bring to boiling; reduce heat. Simmer, uncovered, about 15 minutes or until liquid is reduced to ¼ cup.

3. Add clam juice. Return to boiling; reduce heat. Simmer, uncovered, about 15 minutes more or until liquid is reduced to ¾ cup. Add the asparagus. Cover and cook about 3 minutes or until asparagus is crisp-tender. Stir in tomatoes, parsley, and lemon juice. Season to taste with kosher salt and pepper. Transfer to a serving platter and keep warm.

4. In the same skillet heat the remaining 1 tablespoon olive oil over medium heat. Add salmon; cook for 4 to 6 minutes per ½ inch thickness of salmon or until salmon flakes easily when tested with a fork, turning once. Serve salmon over vegetable mixture. If desired, garnish with fresh thyme.

Nutrition facts per serving: 371 cal., 20 g total fat (4 g sat. fat), 67 mg chol., 289 mg sodium, 12 g carbo., 3 g fiber, 28 g pro.
Exchanges: 1½ Vegetable, ½ Other Carbo., 3½ Lean Meat, 2½ Fat

For Wave 1, serve with cooked quinoa. For Waves 2 and 3, serve with cooked quinoa and red grapes.

Wine Pairing: Sauvignon Blanc

SONOMA SALMON BURGERS

A rich source of iron and vitamins A and C, arugula can now be found in many American supermarkets. Because arugula is a highly perishable leafy green, it should be used quickly and refrigerated for no more than two days.

Prep: 25 minutes **Grill:** 8 minutes **Makes:** 4 servings

1 pound fresh or frozen skinless, boneless salmon fillets

¾ cup sliced pitted ripe olives

¼ cup chopped green onions

1 tablespoon chopped fresh dill

2 teaspoons finely shredded lemon peel

½ teaspoon kosher salt

1 tablespoon extra-virgin olive oil

1½ cups lightly packed arugula leaves

¼ cup thinly sliced celery

1 medium shallot, thinly sliced

2 tablespoons lemon juice

2 large whole wheat pita bread rounds, halved crosswise

Lemon wedges (optional)

Olive Oil

Whole Grains

1. Thaw salmon, if frozen. Rinse salmon; pat dry with paper towels.

2. Cut salmon into pieces. Place salmon in food processor. Cover and pulse with several on-off turns until salmon is coarsely ground. Transfer salmon to a large bowl. Add olives, green onions, dill, lemon peel, and kosher salt to salmon; mix well. Shape salmon mixture into four ½-inch-thick patties. Brush both sides of each salmon patty with olive oil.

3. For a charcoal grill, place salmon patties on the rack of an uncovered grill directly over medium-hot coals. Grill for 8 to 12 minutes or until golden brown, carefully turning once halfway through grilling. (For a gas grill, preheat grill. Reduce heat to medium-high. Place salmon patties on grill rack over heat. Cover and grill as above.)

4. Meanwhile, in a small bowl combine arugula, celery, shallot, and lemon juice. Set aside.

5. Open each pita half to form a pocket. Place one salmon burger and one-fourth of the arugula mixture in each pita half. If desired, serve with lemon wedges.

Nutrition facts per serving: 362 cal., 19 g total fat (3 g sat. fat), 67 mg chol., 708 mg sodium, 22 g carbo., 4 g fiber, 26 g pro.
Exchanges: ½ Vegetable, 1 Starch, 3 Lean Meat, 2 Fat

For Wave 1, serve with cherry tomatoes. For Waves 2 and 3, serve with fresh watermelon.

Wine Pairing: Zinfandel

SONOMA express ROASTED SALMON AND TOMATOES

The flavors of Dijon mustard and marjoram bring a Mediterranean feel to this savory salmon entrée. Salmon fillets are a delicious way to enjoy essential omega-3 fatty acids, which may improve your heart health and lower levels of bad cholesterol while increasing good cholesterol levels.

Prep: 15 minutes **Bake:** 12 minutes **Oven:** 450°F **Makes:** 4 servings

1   1¼-pound fresh or frozen salmon fillet, about 1 inch thick

⅛   teaspoon kosher salt

Nonstick olive oil cooking spray

6   roma tomatoes, seeded and chopped (about 1 pound)

1   tablespoon Worcestershire sauce for chicken

¼   teaspoon coarsely ground black pepper

⅛   teaspoon kosher salt

1   tablespoon Dijon-style mustard

1   tablespoon chopped fresh marjoram or oregano

Fresh oregano sprigs (optional)

Olive Oil

Tomatoes

1. Preheat oven to 450°F. Thaw fish, if frozen. Rinse fish; pat dry with paper towels. Cut fish into four serving-size pieces. Sprinkle with ⅛ teaspoon kosher salt.

2. Lightly coat a 13×9×2-inch baking pan with nonstick cooking spray. Place fish pieces, skin sides up, in prepared pan, tucking under any thin edges. Arrange tomatoes around salmon. Sprinkle tomatoes with Worcestershire sauce, pepper, and ⅛ teaspoon kosher salt. Bake for 12 to 16 minutes or until fish flakes easily when tested with a fork.

3. Remove skin from fish pieces; discard skin. Transfer fish to four dinner plates. Stir mustard and chopped marjoram into tomatoes. Serve tomato mixture with fish. If desired, garnish with oregano sprigs.

Nutrition facts per serving: 283 cal., 15 g total fat (3 g sat. fat), 83 mg chol., 359 mg sodium, 6 g carbo., 1 g fiber, 30 g pro.
Exchanges: 1 Vegetable, 4 Lean Meat, 1 Fat

For Wave 1, serve with Roasted Green Beans with Dried Tomatoes, Goat Cheese, and Olives (page 212) and a whole grain roll. For Waves 2 and 3, serve with Wine Country Grain Medley (page 220) and kiwifruit.

Wine Pairing: Sangiovese

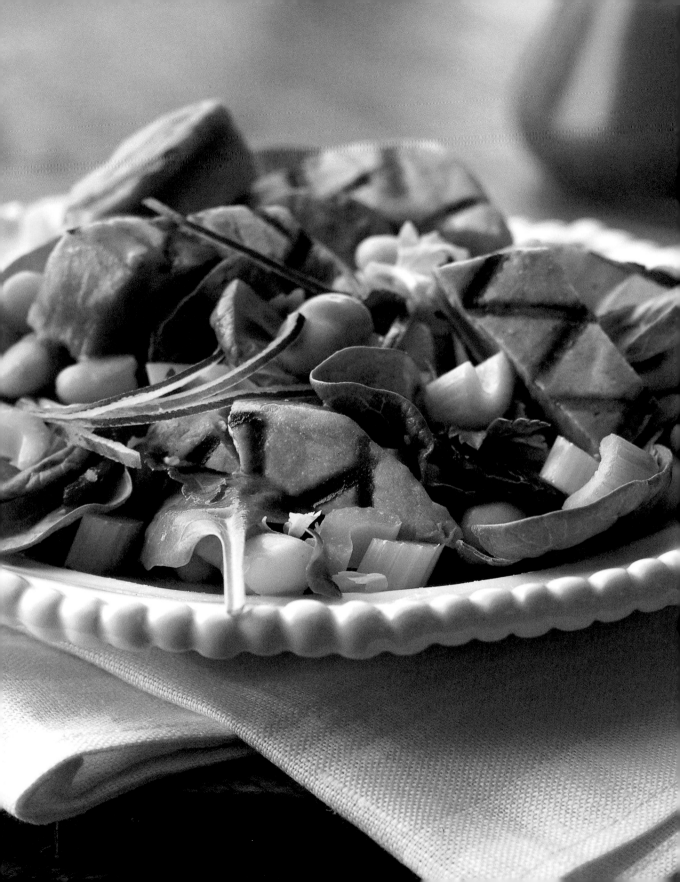

GRILLED TUNA AND CANNELLINI BEAN SALAD

*A no fuss spinach and cannellini bean salad perfectly accompanies grilled tuna steaks
to become a nutritious meal. If you don't have cannellini beans stocked in your
pantry, you can substitute another white bean variety.*

Prep: 25 minutes **Grill:** 8 minutes **Makes:** 4 servings

- 2 5- to 6-ounce fresh or frozen tuna steaks, cut 1 inch thick
- 2 tablespoons lemon juice
- 2 tablespoons extra-virgin olive oil
- 1 tablespoon balsamic vinegar
- 1 tablespoon Dijon-style mustard
- 4 cups fresh baby spinach leaves
- 2 15-ounce cans cannellini beans (white kidney beans), rinsed and drained
- 1 cup thinly sliced red onion
- 1 cup sliced celery
- ¼ cup oil-packed dried tomatoes, drained and chopped
- 2 tablespoons chopped fresh flat-leaf parsley

Olive Oil

Tomatoes

Spinach

1. Thaw fish, if frozen. Rinse fish; pat dry with paper towels. For a charcoal grill, place fish on the greased rack of an uncovered grill directly over medium coals. Grill for 8 to 12 minutes or until fish flakes easily when tested with a fork, gently turning once halfway through grilling. (For a gas grill, preheat grill. Reduce heat to medium. Place fish on greased grill rack over heat. Cover and grill as above.)

2. Meanwhile, for dressing, in a screw-top jar combine lemon juice, olive oil, balsamic vinegar, and Dijon mustard. Cover and shake well. Set aside 1 tablespoon of the dressing to drizzle over grilled fish.

3. In a large bowl combine spinach, beans, red onion, celery, tomatoes, and parsley. Drizzle with remaining dressing; toss gently to coat.

4. To serve, arrange spinach mixture on a serving platter. Slice tuna; place on top of spinach mixture. Drizzle fish with reserved dressing.

Nutrition facts per serving: 306 cal., 9 g total fat (1 g sat. fat), 32 mg chol., 515 mg sodium, 38 g carbo., 12 g fiber, 31 g pro.
Exchanges: 2 Vegetable, 1½ Starch, 3 Very Lean Meat, 1 Fat

For Wave 1, decrease cannellini beans to one 15-ounce can. For Waves 2 and 3, serve with fresh strawberries.

Wine Pairing: Sauvignon Blanc

BROILED TUNA WITH ROSEMARY

Firm-fleshed tuna already has rich flavor. Here rosemary contributes a lemony pine accent for increased flavor dimension.

Prep: 10 minutes **Broil:** 8 minutes **Makes:** 4 servings

4 4-ounce fresh or frozen tuna, halibut, or salmon steaks, cut ½ to 1 inch thick

2 teaspoons extra-virgin olive oil

2 teaspoons lemon juice

⅛ teaspoon kosher salt

⅛ teaspoon freshly ground black pepper

2 cloves garlic, minced (1 teaspoon minced)

2 teaspoons chopped fresh rosemary or tarragon or 1 teaspoon dried herb, crushed

1 tablespoon drained capers, slightly crushed

Olive Oil

1. Preheat broiler. Thaw fish, if frozen. Rinse fish; pat dry with paper towels. Measure thickness of fish. Brush fish with olive oil and lemon juice; season with kosher salt and pepper. Rub garlic and rosemary onto fish.

2. Place fish on the greased rack of an unheated broiler pan. Broil 4 inches from the heat for 4 to 6 minutes per ½-inch thickness of fish or until fish flakes easily when tested with a fork. To serve, top with capers.

Nutrition facts per serving: 145 cal., 3 g total fat (1 g sat. fat), 51 mg chol., 166 mg sodium, 1 g carbo., 0 g fiber, 27 g pro.
Exchanges: 4 Very Lean Meat

For Wave 1, serve with cooked multigrain pasta and cooked eggplant. For Waves 2 and 3, serve with cooked multigrain pasta, Artichoke Salad (page 213), and fresh strawberries.

Wine Pairing: Chardonnay

SNAPPER ON A BED OF FENNEL, CELERY, AND TOMATOES

Snapper is an excellent source of tryptophan, selenium, and vitamin B$_{12}$. Its mild taste contrasts with the licorice flavor of fennel and sweetness of tomatoes to bring you a dish with amazing flavor diversity.

Start to Finish: 40 minutes **Makes:** 4 servings

1   pound fresh or frozen skinless, boneless snapper fillets

    Kosher salt

    Freshly ground black pepper

1   tablespoon extra-virgin olive oil

3   cups thinly sliced fennel

1   cup sliced celery

½   cup sliced onion

6   cloves garlic, minced (1 tablespoon minced)

1   tablespoon chopped fresh thyme

½   cup dry white wine

¼   cup water

½   teaspoon kosher salt

    Dash freshly ground black pepper

1   cup cherry tomatoes, halved

2   tablespoons chopped fresh flat-leaf parsley

1. Thaw fish, if frozen. Rinse fish; pat dry with paper towels. Measure thickness of fish. Season fish with kosher salt and pepper. In a large skillet heat oil over medium-high heat. Add fish; cook about 4 minutes per ½-inch thickness of fish or until fish flakes easily when tested with a fork, turning once halfway through cooking. Remove fish from skillet. Cover and keep warm.

2. Add fennel, celery, onion, garlic, and thyme to skillet. Cover and cook for 5 minutes, stirring occasionally. Add white wine and the water. Bring to boiling; reduce heat. Simmer, uncovered, about 8 minutes or until vegetables are crisp-tender and liquid is slightly reduced. Season with the ½ teaspoon kosher salt and the dash pepper.

3. Stir in tomatoes; place the fish fillets on top of vegetables. Cover and cook for 1 minute to heat through. Sprinkle with parsley.

Nutrition facts per serving: 211 cal., 5 g total fat (1 g sat. fat), 41 mg chol., 499 mg sodium, 11 g carbo., 4 g fiber, 25 g pro.
Exchanges: 2 Vegetable, 3 Very Lean Meat, 1 Fat

For Wave 1, serve with whole grain bread and a mixed green salad. For Waves 2 and 3, serve with whole grain bread and fresh pineapple.

Wine Pairing: Chardonnay

Olive Oil

Tomatoes

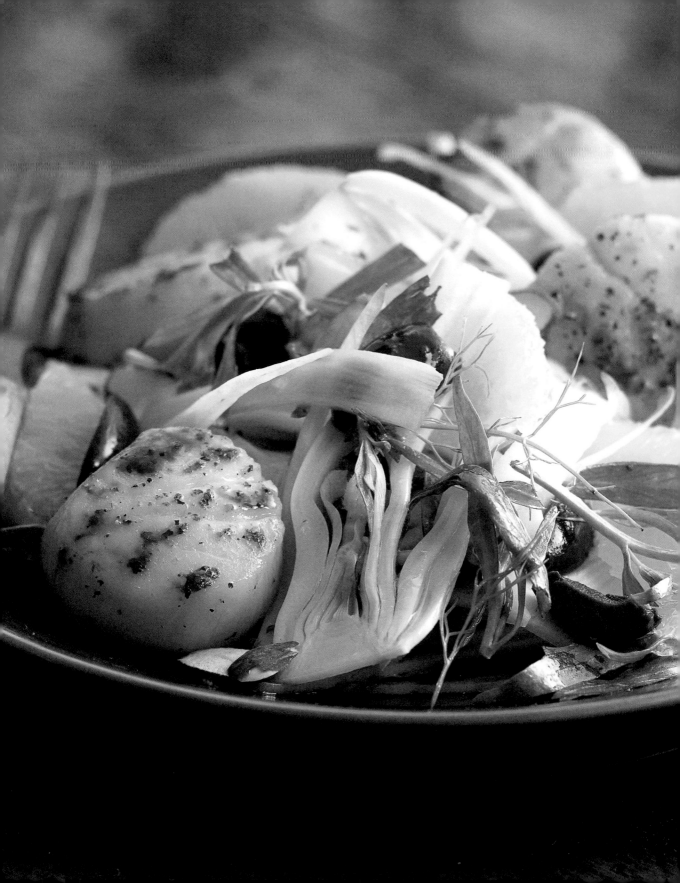

GRILLED SCALLOPS ON FENNEL SLAW

Champagne vinegar is a very light and mild vinegar, ideal for delicate dressings. If you cannot find Champagne vinegar, you can substitute white wine or rice vinegar, but neither will be quite as mild.

Prep: 20 minutes **Grill:** 5 minutes **Makes:** 4 servings

12 fresh or frozen sea scallops
    (1 to 1½ pounds total)

2 medium fennel bulbs

3 medium oranges, peeled and sectioned

¾ cup pitted ripe olives, quartered

⅓ cup chopped fresh tarragon

3 tablespoons lemon juice

2 tablespoons extra-virgin olive oil

1 tablespoon Champagne vinegar

½ teaspoon kosher salt

½ teaspoon freshly ground black pepper

¼ cup sliced almonds, toasted

   Fresh tarragon (optional)

1. Thaw scallops, if frozen. Rinse scallops; pat dry with paper towels. Set aside. If desired, reserve some of the feathery tops from fennel for garnish. Cut off and discard upper stalks from fennel bulbs. Remove any wilted outer layers and cut and discard a thin slice from each fennel base. Cut fennel bulbs into very thin slices.°

2. In a large bowl combine fennel, oranges, olives, tarragon, lemon juice, 1 tablespoon of the olive oil, and the champagne vinegar. Stir in ¼ teaspoon of the kosher salt and ¼ teaspoon of the pepper. Cover and let stand for 15 minutes.

3. Meanwhile, in a large bowl toss scallops with remaining 1 tablespoon olive oil, remaining ¼ teaspoon kosher salt, and remaining ¼ teaspoon pepper. Thread scallops onto long skewers,°° leaving a ¼-inch space between scallops.

4. For a charcoal grill, place skewers on the rack of an uncovered grill directly over medium coals. Grill for 5 to 8 minutes or until scallops are opaque, turning once halfway through grilling. (For a gas grill, preheat grill. Reduce heat to medium. Place skewers on grill rack over heat. Cover and grill as above.)

5. Divide fennel mixture among four dinner plates. Top with scallops; sprinkle with almonds. If desired, garnish with tarragon and/or reserved feathery tops from fennel.

Nutrition facts per serving: 327 cal., 15 g total fat (2 g sat. fat), 37 mg chol., 705 mg sodium, 28 g carbo., 8 g fiber, 24 g pro.
Exchanges: 1½ Vegetable, 1 Fruit, 3 Very Lean Meat, 3 Fat

Broiling directions: Preheat broiler. Place skewers on the unheated rack of a broiler pan. Broil 4 inches from the heat about 8 minutes or until scallops are opaque, turning once halfway through broiling.

*Tip: Use a mandoline to slice fennel very thinly.

**Note: If using wooden skewers, soak in enough water to cover for 1 hour before using.

For Wave 1, this is not appropriate. For Waves 2 and 3, serve with whole grain bread.

Wine Pairing: Sauvignon Blanc

Olive Oil

Almonds

SCALLOPS WITH TROPICAL SALSA

Sweet-tart bursts of papaya enliven this dish of succulent scallops. Scallops are low in fat and offer an excellent source of tryptophan, but because of their delicacy, be cautious not to overcook them or they will toughen and lose their subtle texture.

Start to Finish: 25 minutes **Makes:** 4 servings

1	cup finely chopped papaya or mango
½	cup seeded and chopped red bell pepper
½	cup finely chopped, seeded cucumber
2	tablespoons chopped fresh cilantro
1	fresh jalapeño chile pepper, seeded and finely chopped*
4	teaspoons lime juice
1	teaspoon extra-virgin olive oil
12	ounces fresh or frozen scallops
	Kosher salt
	Freshly ground black pepper
2	teaspoons extra-virgin olive oil
1	clove garlic, minced (½ teaspoon minced)
	Lime wedges (optional)

1. For salsa, in a small bowl stir together the papaya, bell pepper, cucumber, cilantro, chile pepper, lime juice, and olive oil. Let stand at room temperature for at least 15 minutes to allow flavors to blend.

2. Meanwhile, thaw scallops, if frozen. Rinse scallops; pat dry with paper towels. Halve any large scallops. Season scallops lightly with kosher salt and black pepper.

3. In a large nonstick skillet heat olive oil over medium heat. Add garlic; cook for 30 seconds. Add scallops. Cook and stir for 2 to 3 minutes or until scallops are opaque. Use a slotted spoon to remove scallops; drain on paper towels. Serve the scallops with the salsa. If desired, serve with lime wedges.

Nutrition facts per serving: 134 cal., 4 g total fat (1 g sat. fat), 28 mg chol., 262 mg sodium, 9 g carbo., 1 g fiber, 15 g pro.
Exchanges: ½ Fruit, 2½ Very Lean Meat, ½ Fat

*See note, page 76

Olive Oil

Bell Peppers

For Wave 1, this is not appropriate. For Waves 2 and 3, serve with cooked brown rice, steamed asparagus, and fresh grapes.

Wine Pairing: sparkling semisweet

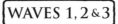

SAUTÉED SHRIMP WITH TOMATO AND BASIL

A bed of nutrient-packed spinach sets the stage for America's favorite shellfish.
Shrimp may be small, but they have huge appeal, especially when
combined with cooked tomatoes, onions, and basil.

Start to Finish: 25 minutes **Makes:** 4 servings

1 pound fresh or frozen medium shrimp

1 tablespoon extra-virgin olive oil

½ cup thinly sliced red onion

3 cups cherry tomatoes, halved

¼ cup chopped fresh basil

3 tablespoons balsamic vinegar

Kosher salt

Freshly ground black pepper

4 cups fresh baby spinach

1. Thaw shrimp, if frozen. Peel and devein shrimp. Rinse shrimp; pat dry with paper towels. In a large skillet heat olive oil over medium-high heat. Add shrimp; cook about 3 minutes or until shrimp are opaque, turning occasionally. Remove shrimp from skillet; set aside.

2. Add red onion to skillet; cook about 3 minutes or until crisp-tender, stirring occasionally. Add tomatoes; cook for 1 minute more. Return shrimp to skillet. Add basil and vinegar; heat through. Season to taste with kosher salt and pepper.

3. Divide spinach among four dinner plates. Top with shrimp mixture.

Nutrition facts per serving: 196 cal., 6 g total fat (1 g sat. fat), 172 mg chol., 319 mg sodium, 11 g carbo., 3 g fiber, 25 g pro.
Exchanges: 2 Vegetable, 3 Very Lean Meat, 1 Fat

For Wave 1, serve with cooked barley. For Waves 2 and 3, serve with cooked barley and fresh mango slices.

Wine Pairing: Zinfandel or Sangiovese

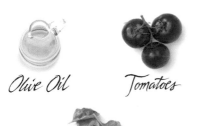

Olive Oil   *Tomatoes*

Spinach

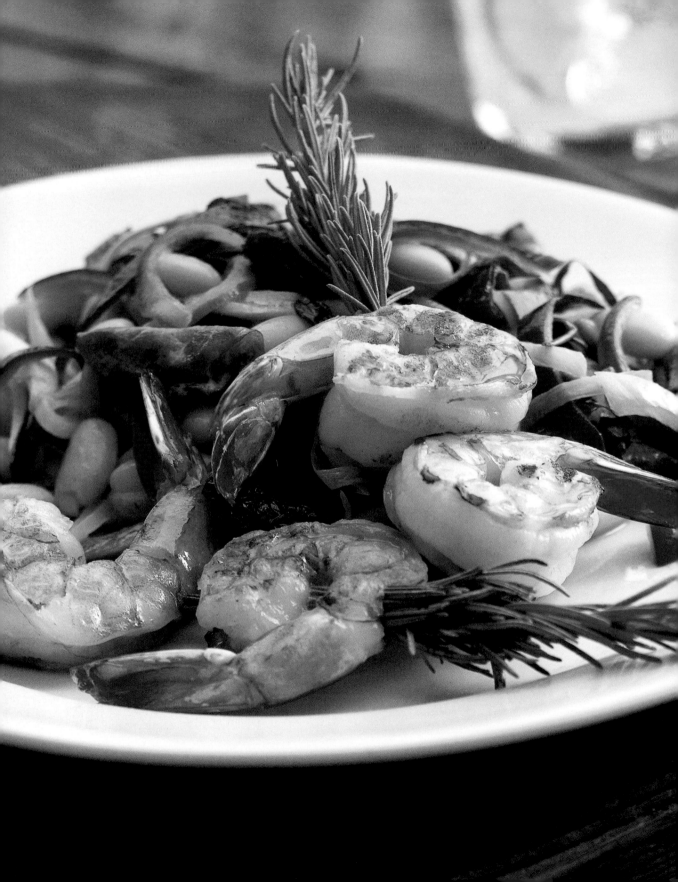

GRILLED SHRIMP WITH WHITE BEANS, ROSEMARY, AND ARUGULA

To devein your shrimp, make a shallow slit along the center of the back and remove the vein by simply washing it out under cold water. These skewered shrimp are grilled in mere minutes with no hassle.

Prep: 30 minutes **Grill:** 8 minutes **Makes:** 4 servings

16 fresh or frozen extra-large shrimp in shells (about 1 pound total)

3 tablespoons extra-virgin olive oil

4 cloves garlic, minced (2 teaspoons minced)

4 teaspoons chopped fresh rosemary

6 cloves garlic, thinly sliced

¼ teaspoon crushed red pepper

¼ teaspoon kosher salt

¼ teaspoon freshly ground black pepper

1 teaspoon finely shredded lemon peel

¼ cup lemon juice

2 tablespoons oil-packed dried tomatoes, drained and finely chopped

2 tablespoons chopped fresh flat-leaf parsley

8 cups lightly packed arugula leaves, fresh spinach, and/or watercress, tough stems removed

1 15-ounce can cannellini beans (white kidney beans), rinsed and drained

½ cup thinly sliced red onion

8 long sprigs fresh rosemary (optional)

1. Thaw shrimp, if frozen. Peel and devein shrimp, leaving tails intact. Thread shrimp onto four 8-inch skewers,° leaving a ¼-inch space between pieces. In a small bowl combine 1 tablespoon of the olive oil, the minced garlic, and 1 teaspoon of the rosemary. Brush all of the oil mixture over shrimp on skewers.

2. For a charcoal grill, place skewers on the rack of an uncovered grill directly over medium coals. Grill about 8 minutes or until shrimp are opaque,

turning once halfway through grilling. (For a gas grill, preheat grill. Reduce heat to medium. Place skewers on grill rack over heat. Cover and grill as above.)

3. Meanwhile, in a very large skillet combine the remaining 2 tablespoons oil, the remaining 1 tablespoon rosemary, the sliced garlic, crushed red pepper, kosher salt, and black pepper. Cook over medium-low heat about 8 minutes or until garlic is lightly browned, stirring occasionally. Stir in lemon peel, lemon juice, tomatoes, and parsley.

4. Add half of the arugula, the beans, and onion to mixture in skillet. Cook, tossing constantly, just until arugula begins to wilt. Add the remaining arugula; cook, tossing constantly, about 1 minute more or just until arugula is wilted.

5. Divide arugula mixture among four dinner plates. If desired, remove shrimp from wooden skewers and skewer two shrimp on each rosemary sprig. Serve shrimp with arugula mixture.

Nutrition facts per serving: 311 cal., 13 g total fat (2 g sat. fat), 172 mg chol., 477 mg sodium, 23 g carbo., 6 g fiber, 31 g pro.
Exchanges: 2 Vegetable, 1 Starch, 3 Very Lean Meat, 2 Fat

*Note: If using wooden skewers, soak in enough water to cover for at least 1 hour before grilling.

For Wave 1, serve with whole grain bread. For Waves 2 and 3, serve with whole grain bread and cantaloupe.

Wine Pairing: Sauvignon Blanc

Olive Oil

Tomatoes

Spinach

STEAMED CLAMS WITH GARLIC, WHITE BEANS, AND GREENS

Garlic enthusiasts will relish this dish. Twenty garlic cloves may sound like a lot, but their flavor becomes less intense with cooking. You can save yourself a lot of time and still enjoy the same wonderful flavor by using 3 tablespoons of bottled minced garlic.

Start to Finish: 40 minutes **Makes:** 4 servings

2 tablespoons extra-virgin olive oil

½ cup thinly sliced garlic cloves (about 2 bulbs or 20 cloves)*

1 cup thinly sliced red onion

2 pounds Manila or other clams in shells, rinsed well (about 20)

½ cup dry white wine

1 tablespoon chopped fresh oregano

4 cups Swiss chard, stemmed and cut into 1-inch-wide strips

1 cup chopped tomato

1 cup canned cannellini beans (white kidney beans)

Kosher salt

Freshly ground black pepper

Lemon wedges

Olive Oil

Tomatoes

1. In a 4-quart Dutch oven heat oil over low heat. Add the garlic; cook about 5 minutes or until translucent with no color. Add the red onion and cook for 5 minutes more. Add the clams, white wine, and oregano. Bring to boiling; reduce heat. Cover and simmer for 5 to 10 minutes or until the clams open. Remove the clams from the Dutch oven as they open; discard any that do not open.

2. Add Swiss chard, tomato, and white beans to liquid in Dutch oven. Cook about 3 minutes or until chard wilts. Season to taste with kosher salt and pepper.

3. Divide the chard mixture among four shallow serving bowls. Top with clams. Serve with lemon wedges.

Nutrition facts per serving: 254 cal., 8 g total fat (1 g sat. fat), 36 mg chol., 375 mg sodium, 25 g carbo., 5 g fiber, 20 g pro.
Exchanges: 1½ Vegetable, 1 Starch, 2 Very Lean Meat, 1½ Fat

*Note: To cut prep time, omit the sliced garlic and use 3 tablespoons bottled minced garlic.

For Wave 1, serve with steamed asparagus. For Waves 2 and 3, serve with fresh grapefruit.

Wine Pairing: Sauvignon Blanc

SESAME CRAB AND BROWN RICE CAKES

This burger-style recipe calls for lump crabmeat, which has large, choice chunks of meat from the body of the crab. When combined with these Asian ingredients, this burger becomes a mouthwatering delicacy.

Prep: 30 minutes **Cook:** 10 minutes per batch **Makes:** 6 servings (2 cakes per serving)

1 tablespoon reduced-sodium soy sauce

1 tablespoon seasoned rice vinegar

2 to 3 teaspoons bottled hot pepper sauce (optional)

2 teaspoons honey

2 teaspoons sweet rice wine (mirin)

1 teaspoon toasted sesame oil

¼ teaspoon kosher salt

1 egg

¼ cup chopped green onions

2 tablespoons sesame seeds, toasted

2 tablespoons chopped fresh cilantro

1 pound cooked crabmeat, flaked, or three 6½-ounce cans lump crabmeat, drained, flaked, and cartilage removed

3 cups cooked brown rice, cooled

1 to 2 tablespoons canola oil

½ cup Miso Vinaigrette

Whole Grains

1. In a large bowl whisk together soy sauce, rice vinegar, hot pepper sauce (if desired), honey, rice wine, sesame oil, and kosher salt. Add egg; whisk lightly to combine. Stir in green onions, sesame seeds, and cilantro. Add crabmeat and cooked rice. Mix well. Form crab mixture into twelve 1-inch thick patties, using about ½ cup mixture for each patty.

2. In a large nonstick skillet heat 1 tablespoon of the canola oil over medium heat. Cook patties, in batches, in hot oil about 10 minutes or until an instant-read thermometer inserted in the center of each patty registers 160°F; turn patties once. If necessary to prevent overbrowning, reduce heat to medium-low. (Add additional canola oil as needed during cooking.) Serve with Miso Vinaigrette.

Nutrition facts per serving: 331 cal., 14 g total fat (2 g sat. fat), 75 mg chol., 1293 mg sodium, 30 g carbo., 3 g fiber, 20 g pro.
Exchanges: 1½ Starch, ½ Other Carbo., 2½ Very Lean Meat, 2 Fat

Miso Vinaigrette: In a blender combine ¼ cup red miso, ¼ cup seasoned rice vinegar, ¼ cup peanut oil, 2 tablespoons toasted sesame oil, 1 tablespoon honey, 1 tablespoon reduced-sodium soy sauce, and ½ teaspoon grated fresh ginger. Cover and blend until smooth. Pour into an airtight container; cover and store in the refrigerator for up to 1 week. Makes about 1 cup.

For Wave 1, this is not appropriate. For Waves 2 and 3, serve with steamed bok choy or green cabbage and orange slices.

Wine Pairing: Zinfandel

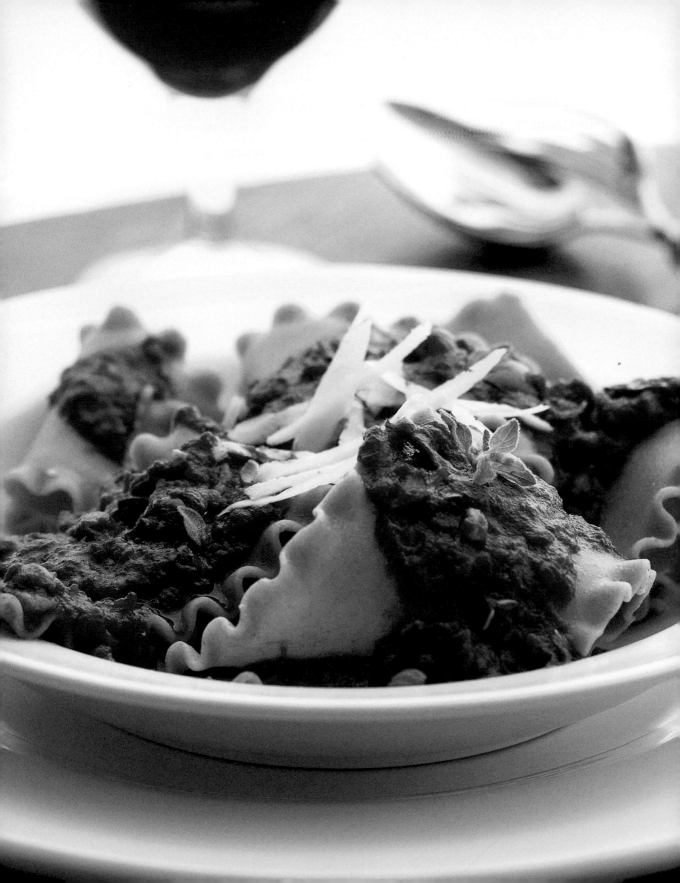

Meatless Meals

There's no shortage of alternatives to meat and fish for the protein portion of your Sonoma Diet plate, as the following meal ideas confirm. And you don't need to be a vegetarian to enjoy the delicious and surprisingly satisfying meatless dishes in this chapter. In fact, not all of them are strictly for protein. You'll also find recipes here with generous offerings of whole grains and vegetables.

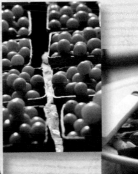

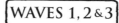

SPAGHETTI WITH ROASTED TOMATOES AND PINE NUTS

This earthy Italian recipe presents like a gourmet dish. Toasted pine nuts add crunch and nuttiness; be sure to stir them frequently while toasting because they burn easily if unattended.

Prep: 20 minutes **Bake:** 10 minutes **Oven:** 400°F **Makes:** 4 servings

6 ounces dried multigrain spaghetti (such as Barilla Plus)

2 cups cherry tomatoes, halved

¼ cup extra-virgin olive oil

¼ teaspoon kosher salt

⅛ teaspoon freshly ground black pepper

3 cloves garlic, minced (1½ teaspoons minced)

¼ to ½ teaspoon crushed red pepper

1 15-ounce can cannellini beans (white kidney beans), rinsed and drained

6 cups fresh baby spinach leaves

1 cup chopped fresh basil

1 teaspoon lemon juice

¼ cup pine nuts, toasted

¼ cup shredded Parmesan cheese (1 ounce)

1. Preheat oven to 400°F. Cook spaghetti according to package directions; drain. Return to hot pan; cover and keep warm. Meanwhile, place tomatoes in a 15×10×1-inch baking pan. Drizzle tomatoes with 2 tablespoons of the olive oil; sprinkle with the kosher salt and pepper. Toss gently to coat. Bake about 10 minutes or until tender.

2. Meanwhile, in a medium skillet heat the remaining 2 tablespoons olive oil over medium heat. Add garlic and crushed red pepper; cook about 30 seconds or just until fragrant. Stir in cannellini beans; heat through.

3. Place tomatoes in a large serving bowl. Top with baby spinach, basil, lemon juice, bean mixture, and cooked pasta. Toss to combine. Top individual servings with pine nuts and Parmesan cheese.

Nutrition facts per serving: 435 cal., 21 g total fat (4 g sat. fat), 4 mg chol., 430 mg sodium, 51 g carbo., 10 g fiber, 20 g pro.
Exchanges: 2 Vegetable, 2½ Starch, 1½ Very Lean Meat, 3 Fat

For Wave 1, serve as is. For Waves 2 and 3, serve with fresh grapes.

Wine Pairing: Burgundy or Sangiovese

Olive Oil

Tomatoes

Spinach

Whole Grains

EGGPLANT AND CAPER TOMATO SAUCE

A flavorful blend of capers, kalamata olives, basil, and thyme fills this dish with flavors of typical Mediterranean cuisine. The meaty flesh of the eggplant is very filling but contains very few calories and little fat, making it a perfect vegetarian main-dish option.

Prep: 30 minutes **Bake:** 18 minutes **Cook:** 10 minutes + 15 minutes **Oven:** 375°F **Makes:** 8 servings

1 medium eggplant, peeled and cut into 1-inch cubes (about 1 pound)

¼ cup extra-virgin olive oil

1 large onion, chopped

6 cloves garlic, minced (1 tablespoon minced)

3 pounds tomatoes, cored and chopped, or four 14½-ounce cans diced tomatoes, undrained

½ cup capers, rinsed and drained

½ cup pitted kalamata olives, coarsely chopped

2 tablespoons chopped fresh basil

1 tablespoon chopped fresh oregano

1 tablespoon chopped fresh thyme

Kosher salt

Freshly ground black pepper

12 ounces dried multigrain spaghetti (such as Barilla Plus)

¼ cup finely shredded Parmesan cheese (2 ounces)

1. Preheat oven to 375°F. Place eggplant cubes in a 15×10×1-inch baking pan. Drizzle eggplant with 2 tablespoons of the olive oil; toss to coat. Bake for 18 to 20 minutes or until eggplant is tender but still holding its shape.

2. Meanwhile, in a large saucepan heat the remaining 2 tablespoons olive oil over medium heat. Add onion; cook for 5 minutes, stirring occasionally. Add eggplant and garlic; cook about 10 minutes more or until eggplant is very soft and starting to break apart, stirring occasionally.

3. Add tomatoes, capers, and olives to eggplant mixture. Bring to boiling; reduce heat. Cover and simmer for 10 minutes, stirring occasionally. Uncover and simmer for 15 to 20 minutes more or until desired consistency, stirring occasionally. Stir in basil, oregano, and thyme. Season to taste with kosher salt and pepper.

4. Meanwhile, cook pasta according to package directions; drain well. Return to hot pan; cover and keep warm. Serve sauce over cooked pasta; sprinkle with cheese.

Nutrition facts per serving: 311 cal., 11 g total fat (2 g sat. fat), 5 mg chol., 559 mg sodium, 43 g carbo., 8 g fiber, 13 g pro.
Exchanges: 2 Vegetable, 2 Starch, 2 Fat

For Wave 1, serve as is. For Waves 2 and 3, serve with fresh berries.

Wine Pairing: Sangiovese

Olive Oil

Tomatoes

Whole Grains

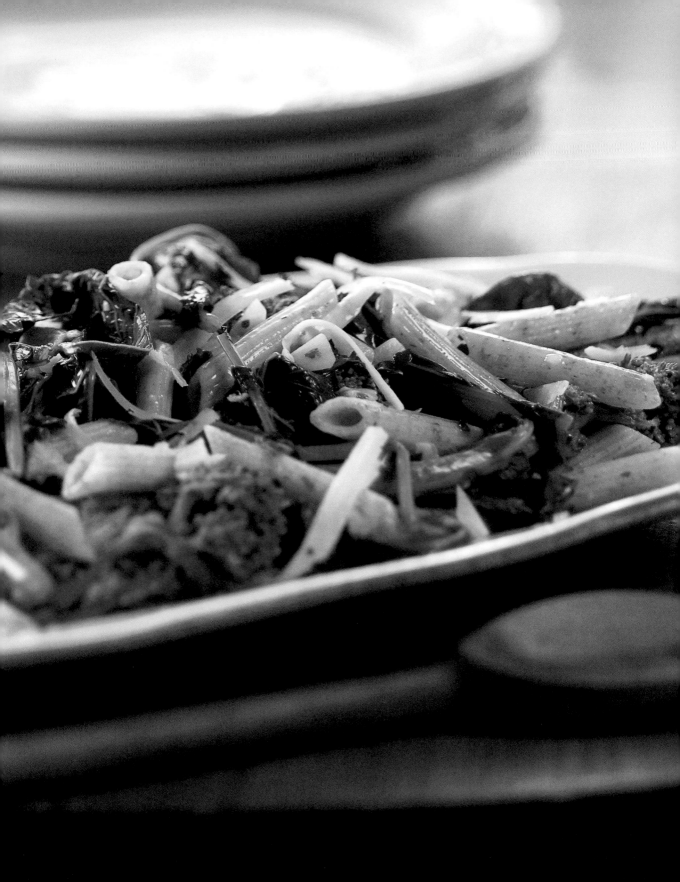

BROCCOLI RAAB AND PENNE

Although it has broccoli in its name, broccoli raab is actually closely related to the cabbage and turnip families. Its pungent, somewhat bitter flavor is mellowed by a short cooking time.

Start to Finish: 25 minutes **Makes:** 6 servings

1 pound broccoli raab

8 ounces dried multigrain penne pasta (such as Barilla Plus)

2 tablespoons extra-virgin olive oil

6 cloves garlic, minced (1 tablespoon minced)

¼ to ½ teaspoon crushed red pepper

¼ cup grated Parmesan cheese

1 tablespoon lemon juice

Kosher salt

Freshly ground black pepper

⅓ cup shredded Parmesan cheese

Olive Oil

Whole Grains

1. Trim tough stems from broccoli raab; discard stems. Coarsely chop the broccoli raab leaves. In a Dutch oven cook broccoli raab in a large amount of salted boiling water for 5 to 7 minutes or until tender. Drain; submerse broccoli raab into a large bowl of ice water to cool quickly. When cool, drain well.

2. Meanwhile, cook pasta according to package directions. Drain pasta, reserving ¾ cup of the cooking water.

3. In a large skillet heat olive oil over medium heat. Add garlic and crushed red pepper; cook for 1 minute. Add drained broccoli raab; toss to coat with oil. Add the drained pasta, reserved pasta cooking water, grated Parmesan cheese, and lemon juice. Cook and stir until heated through. Season to taste with kosher salt and black pepper. Sprinkle each serving with shredded Parmesan cheese.

Nutrition facts per serving: 238 cal., 7 g total fat (2 g sat. fat), 6 mg chol., 263 mg sodium, 30 g carbo., 5 g fiber, 12 g pro.
Exchanges: 1 Vegetable, 2 Starch, ½ Lean Meat, 1 Fat

For Wave 1, serve with bell pepper strips. For Waves 2 and 3, serve with fresh raspberries.

Wine Pairing: Sauvignon Blanc

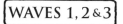
SPAGHETTI WITH FRESH MARINARA

*Fresh tomatoes, garlic, and herbs make a brilliant sauce, like nothing you'll find in a jar.
Enjoy your fresh marinara sauce over multigrain spaghetti.*

Prep: 30 minutes   **Cook:** 20 minutes   **Makes:** 6 servings

3	tablespoons extra-virgin olive oil
1	cup chopped onion
1	cup chopped red bell pepper
12	cloves garlic, minced (2 tablespoons minced)
6	cups chopped roma tomatoes (about 2½ pounds) or four 14½-ounce cans diced tomatoes, undrained
¼	cup tomato paste
10	ounces dried multigrain spaghetti (such as Barilla Plus)
3	tablespoons chopped fresh basil
2	tablespoons chopped fresh oregano
1	tablespoon chopped fresh thyme
½	teaspoon kosher salt
¼	teaspoon freshly ground black pepper
½	cup finely shredded Parmesan cheese (2 ounces)

1. In a large saucepan heat oil over medium heat. Add onion, bell pepper, and garlic; cook for 5 minutes, stirring occasionally. Stir in tomatoes and tomato paste. Bring to boiling; reduce heat. Simmer, uncovered, for 20 minutes.

2. Meanwhile, cook spaghetti according to package directions. Drain well. Return to hot pan; keep warm.

3. Stir basil, oregano, thyme, kosher salt, and black pepper into tomato mixture. Cool slightly. Transfer half of the tomato mixture to a blender or food processor; cover and blend or process until nearly smooth. Repeat with remaining tomato mixture.

4. Return all of the blended tomato mixture to the same saucepan. Heat through. Serve over hot cooked spaghetti. Sprinkle individual servings with Parmesan cheese.

Nutrition facts per serving: 324 cal., 10 g total fat (2 g sat. fat), 5 mg chol., 393 mg sodium, 48 g carbo., 7 g fiber, 14 g pro.
Exchanges: 2 Vegetable, 2½ Starch, ½ Lean Meat, 1 Fat

For Wave 1, serve with a mixed green salad. For Waves 2 and 3, serve with fresh pear slices.

Wine Pairing: Chianti

Olive Oil

Tomatoes

Bell Peppers

Whole Grains

EGGPLANT PARMESAN

Here's a basic, but hearty version of a classic vegetarian dish. The layers of vegetables and cheeses in this eggplant Parmesan are enhanced by a variety of fresh herbs.

Prep: 15 minutes **Bake:** 20 minutes + 30 minutes **Stand:** 10 minutes **Oven:** 375°F **Makes:** 8 servings

Nonstick olive oil cooking spray

2 medium eggplants (about 2 pounds total)

2 tablespoons extra-virgin olive oil

6 cloves garlic, minced (1 tablespoon minced)

3 tablespoons chopped fresh thyme, oregano, and/or marjoram

3 cups purchased marinara sauce

3 tablespoons chopped fresh basil

1½ cups shredded part-skim mozzarella cheese (6 ounces)

½ cup grated Parmesan cheese

Olive Oil

Tomatoes

1. Preheat oven to 375°F. Coat two large baking sheets with nonstick cooking spray; set aside. Trim ends from eggplants and discard. Cut eggplants crosswise into ½-inch-thick slices. Arrange eggplant slices in a single layer on prepared baking sheets. In a small bowl combine olive oil, garlic, and thyme. Drizzle over eggplant slices. Bake for 20 to 25 minutes or until tender but still intact.

2. Coat a 2-quart rectangular baking dish with nonstick cooking spray. In a medium bowl combine marinara sauce and basil. In another medium bowl combine mozzarella cheese and Parmesan cheese. Spread ½ cup of the sauce in the prepared baking dish. Top with one-third of the eggplant slices, overlapping if necessary. Top with one-third of the remaining sauce and one-third of the cheese mixture. Repeat layers twice, starting with eggplant and ending with cheese.

3. Bake, covered, in the 375°F oven about 30 minutes or until heated through. Uncover; let stand for 10 minutes before serving.

Nutrition facts per serving: 196 cal., 11 g total fat (4 g sat. fat), 18 mg chol., 644 mg sodium, 17 g carbo., 6 g fiber, 10 g pro.
Exchanges: 2 Vegetable, ½ Other Carbo., 1 Medium-Fat Meat, 1 Fat

For Wave 1, serve with cooked multigrain pasta. For Waves 2 and 3, serve with cooked multigrain pasta and fresh grapes.

Wine Pairing: Chianti

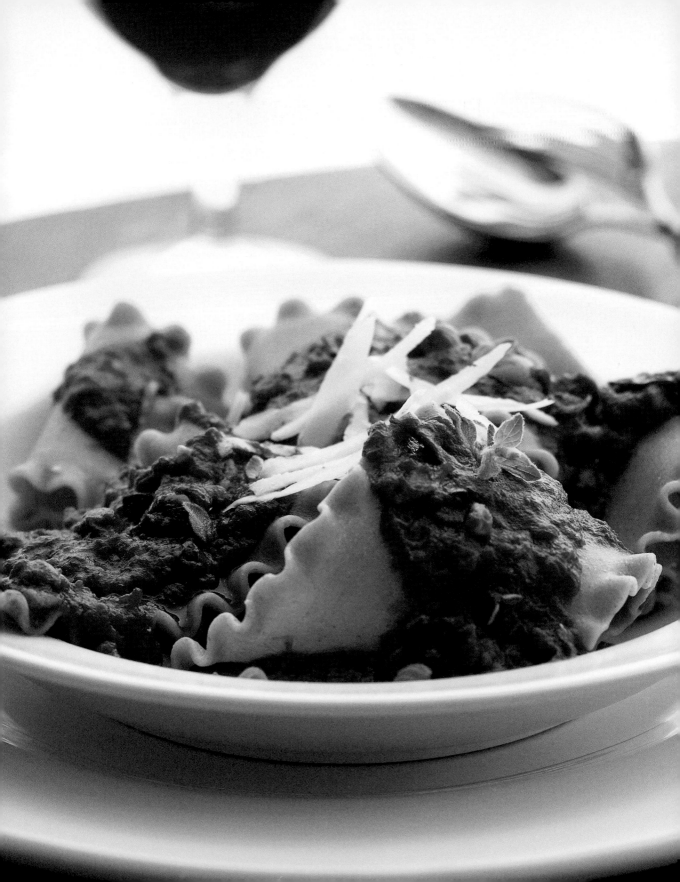

PUTTANESCA SAUCE

This slightly spicy Italian pasta sauce has immense flavor. The last-minute addition of thyme and marjoram lends a warm, minty accent.

Prep: 25 minutes **Cook:** 30 minutes **Makes:** 6 servings

1 tablespoon extra-virgin olive oil

6 cloves garlic, minced
(1 tablespoon minced)

3 14½-ounce cans crushed tomatoes

¼ teaspoon crushed red pepper

¼ cup pitted kalamata olives, chopped

¼ cup capers, rinsed and drained

2 tablespoons balsamic vinegar

¼ teaspoon kosher salt

¼ teaspoon freshly ground black pepper

1 tablespoon chopped fresh thyme

2 teaspoons chopped fresh marjoram

10 ounces dried multigrain pasta, such as lasagna noodles, spaghetti, or fettuccine (such as Barilla Plus)

¼ cup finely shredded Parmesan cheese (1 ounce)

1. In a medium saucepan heat olive oil over medium heat. Add garlic; cook for 30 seconds. Stir in tomatoes and crushed red pepper; bring to boiling.

2. Stir in olives, capers, vinegar, kosher salt, and black pepper. Return to boiling; reduce heat to low. Simmer, uncovered, about 30 minutes or until desired consistency. Stir in thyme and marjoram

3. Meanwhile, cook pasta according to package directions. Drain. Serve sauce over hot cooked pasta. Sprinkle with Parmesan cheese.

Nutrition facts per serving: 296 cal., 6 g total fat (1 g sat. fat), 2 mg chol., 636 mg sodium, 53 g carbo., 7 g fiber, 11 g pro.
Exchanges: 2 Vegetable, 2½ Starch, 1 Fat

For Wave 1, serve with a spinach salad. For Waves 2 and 3, serve with a spinach salad and fresh grapes.

Wine Pairing: Zinfandel

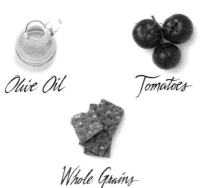

Olive Oil *Tomatoes*

Whole Grains

BARLEY RISOTTO WITH ROASTED SQUASH

Traditional Italian risotto is made with rice, but this nutrient-dense variation uses barley as the grain source. Barley lends a slight nutty flavor and is a very good source of fiber and selenium.

Prep: 40 minutes **Roast:** 30 minutes **Bake:** 8 minutes **Oven:** 400°F **Makes:** 6 servings

1 pound butternut squash, peeled, halved, seeded, and cut in 1-inch pieces

3 tablespoons extra-virgin olive oil

½ teaspoon kosher salt

¼ teaspoon freshly ground black pepper

   Dash ground nutmeg

1 pound regular barley (not quick-cooking) (2 cups), rinsed

6 cups reduced-sodium chicken broth

1 cup finely chopped onion

6 cloves garlic, minced (1 tablespoon minced)

½ cup dry white wine

½ cup finely shredded Parmesan cheese (2 ounces)

1 tablespoon chopped fresh thyme

1 teaspoon chopped fresh sage

1 tablespoon chopped fresh flat-leaf parsley

Olive Oil   *Whole Grains*

1. Preheat oven to 400°F. Place squash in a shallow baking pan. Add 1 tablespoon of the olive oil, the kosher salt, pepper, and nutmeg. Toss to coat. Roast about 30 minutes or until tender. Set aside. Place barley in another shallow baking pan. Bake for 8 to 10 minutes or until lightly toasted; set aside.

2. In a large saucepan heat broth over medium heat just until simmering; reduce heat. Cover and keep warm over low heat.

3. In a 4-quart Dutch oven heat the remaining 2 tablespoons oil over medium heat. Add onion and garlic; cook until onion is tender, stirring occasionally. Stir in toasted barley; cook and stir for 2 minutes. Stir in wine. Cook and stir until wine is absorbed. Add 1 cup of the hot broth; cook, uncovered, until most of the broth is absorbed, stirring frequently. Continue adding broth, 1 cup at a time, cooking after each addition until broth is nearly absorbed, stirring frequently. When the last of the broth has been added, cook until mixture is creamy. (Total cooking time should be 30 to 35 minutes after the wine is added.) Fold in roasted squash, Parmesan cheese, thyme, and sage. Top individual servings with parsley.

Nutrition facts per serving: 435 cal., 10 g total fat (2 g sat. fat), 5 mg chol., 859 mg sodium, 70 g carbo., 15 g fiber, 16 g pro.
Exchanges: 4½ Starch, ½ Lean Meat, 1 Fat

For Wave 1, this is not appropriate. For Waves 2 and 3, serve with a tossed green salad and fresh apple slices.

Wine Pairing: Sauvignon Blanc

SUMMER SQUASH AND CHARD GRATIN

*This scrumptious, cheesy vegetable casserole is perfect for summer months when chard is at its best.
Chard's bitterness is subdued with the sweeter flavors of squash and ricotta cheese.*

Prep: 35 minutes **Bake:** 30 minutes **Stand:** 10 minutes **Oven:** 350°F **Makes:** 6 servings

1 tablespoon extra-virgin olive oil

2 cups chopped onion

6 cloves garlic, minced (1 tablespoon minced)

1 8-ounce package sliced mushrooms (3 cups)

1½ pounds zucchini and/or yellow summer squash, thinly sliced (6 cups)

1 pound Swiss chard, stemmed and coarsely shredded (8 cups)

2 eggs

1 cup part-skim ricotta cheese

1 cup low-fat or fat-free milk

2 ounces Parmesan cheese, finely shredded (½ cup)

2 tablespoons chopped fresh dill

½ teaspoon kosher salt

¼ teaspoon freshly ground black pepper

Olive Oil

1. Preheat oven to 350°F. In a very large skillet heat oil over medium heat. Add onion; cook and stir about 5 minutes or until tender. Stir in garlic; cook for 30 to 60 seconds or until tender. Add mushrooms; cook for 5 to 8 minutes or until lightly browned and no liquid remains.

2. In a large covered saucepan cook zucchini and Swiss chard in a small amount of lightly salted boiling water for 3 to 5 minutes or until crisp-tender. Drain well. Stir zucchini and swiss chard into mushroom mixture. Transfer vegetable mixture to a 2-quart baking dish or au gratin dish; set aside.

3. In a medium bowl slightly beat eggs. Stir in ricotta cheese, milk, Parmesan cheese, dill, kosher salt, and pepper. Spoon egg mixture evenly over vegetables.

4. Bake for 30 to 35 minutes or until set and lightly browned on top (it should jiggle slightly in the middle when gently shaken). Let stand, uncovered, for 10 minutes before serving.

Nutrition facts per serving: 225 cal., 11 g total fat (5 g sat. fat), 92 mg chol., 590 mg sodium, 19 g carbo., 4 g fiber, 16 g pro.
Exchanges: 3 Vegetable, 1½ Lean Meat, 1½ Fat

For Wave 1, serve with cooked bulgur. For Waves 2 and 3, serve with cooked bulgur and fresh kiwifruit.

Wine Pairing: Sauvignon Blanc

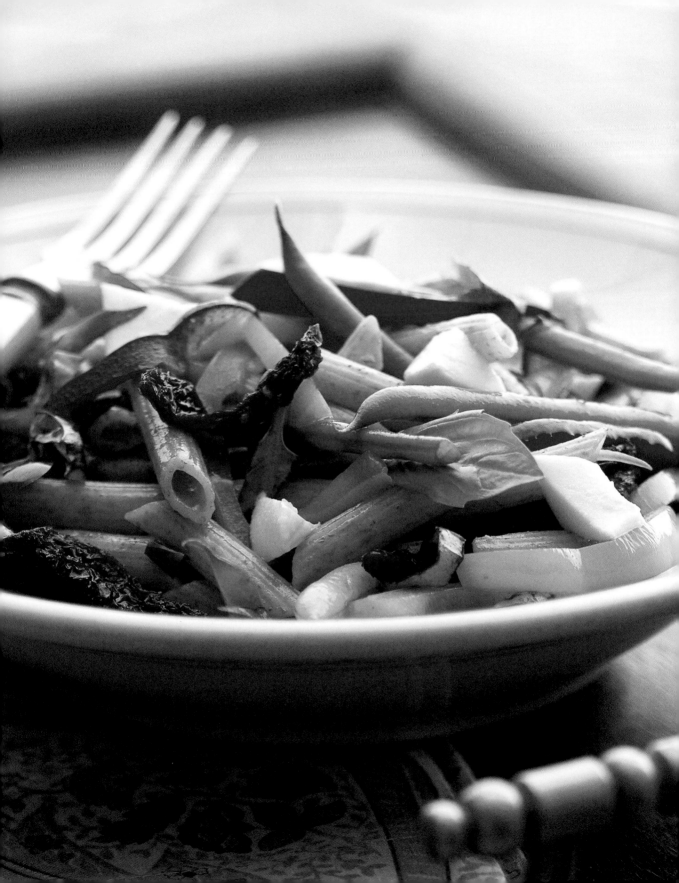

PASTA WITH GREEN BEANS AND DRIED TOMATOES

This summery pasta concoction comes together in no time, and with all those colorful vegetables, you know this dish is full of health and nutrition. Dried tomatoes accent the dish with bursts of sweet-tart flavor.

Start to Finish: 35 minutes **Makes:** 4 servings

4 quarts water

1 tablespoon kosher salt

8 ounces dried multigrain penne (such as Barilla Plus)

12 ounces fresh green beans or 3 cups frozen whole green beans

1 tablespoon extra-virgin olive oil

3 large red and/or yellow bell peppers, seeded and cut into bite-size strips

1 tablespoon bottled minced garlic

¼ cup oil-packed dried tomatoes, drained and cut into ¼-inch-thick slices

2 tablespoons chopped fresh basil, flat-leaf parsley, and/or oregano

3 tablespoons balsamic vinegar

Kosher salt

Freshly ground black pepper

2 ounces fresh mozzarella cheese, cut up

Fresh basil leaves (optional)

1. In a large Dutch oven combine the water and the 1 tablespoon kosher salt; bring to boiling. Add pasta and, if using, fresh beans. Cook according to pasta package directions, adding frozen green beans (if using) for the last 5 minutes of cooking time. Drain pasta and beans, reserving 1 cup of the cooking water.

2. Meanwhile, in a large skillet heat olive oil over medium-high heat. Add pepper strips; cook for 5 minutes, stirring occasionally. Add the garlic; cook for 30 seconds more. Add the dried tomatoes, basil, and drained pasta mixture. Cook, tossing frequently, until heated through. Stir in balsamic vinegar and enough of the reserved pasta liquid to moisten pasta mixture to desired consistency. Season to taste with additional kosher salt and black pepper. Top with cheese cubes. If desired, garnish with fresh basil.

Nutrition facts per serving: 348 cal., 9 g total fat (3 g sat. fat), 11 mg chol., 501 mg sodium, 54 g carbo., 9 g fiber, 16 g pro.
Exchanges: 2 Vegetable, 3 Starch, ½ Medium-Fat Meat, ½ Fat

For Wave 1, serve as is. For Waves 2 and 3, serve with fresh orange slices.

Wine Pairing: Zinfandel

Olive Oil

Tomatoes

Bell Peppers

Whole Grains

CAULIFLOWER AND CHICKPEA GRATIN

A truly unique gratin, this dish features chickpeas, a legume used extensively in Mediterranean cooking. Don't let the labels fool you; chickpeas and garbanzo beans are actually the same thing.

Prep: 30 minutes **Cook:** 15 minutes **Broil:** 1 minute **Makes:** 6 servings

3 tablespoons extra-virgin olive oil

2 cups chopped onion

2 14½-ounce cans diced tomatoes, drained

1 15-ounce can garbanzo beans (chickpeas), rinsed and drained

6 cloves garlic, minced (1 tablespoon minced)

¼ cup chopped fresh flat-leaf parsley

2 tablespoons capers, rinsed and drained

1 tablespoon chopped fresh oregano

1 tablespoon lemon juice

1 teaspoon chopped fresh thyme

½ teaspoon kosher salt

¼ teaspoon freshly ground black pepper

1¾ pounds cauliflower, cut into florets

4 ounces feta cheese, crumbled

1. In a large saucepan heat olive oil over medium-high heat. Add onion; cook about 5 minutes or until tender, stirring occasionally. Add drained tomatoes, garbanzo beans, and garlic. Bring to boiling; reduce heat to low. Cover and simmer for 15 minutes. Stir in parsley, capers, oregano, lemon juice, thyme, kosher salt, and pepper.

2. Meanwhile, in a covered Dutch oven cook cauliflower in a small amount of boiling water about 5 minutes or just until tender. Drain and keep warm.

3. Transfer cauliflower to a 2- to 2½-quart broilerproof baking dish. Top with hot tomato mixture. Sprinkle with feta cheese. Broil 3 to 4 inches from the heat for 1 to 2 minutes or just until cheese begins to brown. Serve immediately.

Nutrition facts per serving: 271 cal., 12 g total fat (4 g sat. fat), 17 mg chol., 951 mg sodium, 35 g carbo., 9 g fiber, 10 g pro.
Exchanges: 3 Vegetable, 1 Starch, 1 Medium-Fat Meat, 1 Fat

For Wave 1, serve as is. For Waves 2 and 3, serve with fresh orange slices.

Wine Pairing: Chardonnay

Olive Oil

Tomatoes

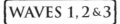

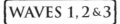

CREPES FILLED WITH MUSHROOMS, SPINACH, AND FRESH MOZZARELLA

It's best to plan ahead for this elegant entrée. Make your crepes beforehand so, come mealtime, you'll only have to make the filling.

Prep: 45 minutes **Broil:** 1 minute **Makes:** 4 servings

1   tablespoon extra-virgin olive oil

1½ pounds assorted fresh mushrooms (such as stemmed shiitake, oyster, or cremini), sliced (about 10 cups)

Kosher salt

Freshly ground black pepper

6   cloves garlic, minced (1 tablespoon)

2   tablespoons balsamic vinegar

2   cups fresh baby spinach

2   ounces fresh mozzarella cheese, cut into ½-inch cubes, or ½ cup shredded part-skim mozzarella cheese (2 ounces)

2   tablespoons chopped fresh basil

1   recipe Basic Crepes or eight 8-inch whole wheat tortillas

¼   cup finely shredded Parmesan cheese (1 ounce)

Nutrition facts per serving: 381 cal., 15 g total fat (5 g sat. fat), 122 mg chol., 485 mg sodium, 51 g carbo., 8 g fiber, 17 g pro.
Exchanges: 3 Vegetable, 2½ Starch, 1 Medium-Fat Meat, 1 Fat

Basic Crepes: In a blender combine 2 eggs; ⅔ cup water; ½ cup low-fat milk; 1 tablespoon extra-virgin olive oil, 1¼ teaspoons fresh flat-leaf parsley, basil or thyme; ¼ teaspoon kosher salt; and ⅛ teaspoon freshly ground black pepper; add 1 cup whole wheat flour. Cover and blend on low speed until combined; blend on high speed for 1 minute. Pour into a medium bowl; cover lightly and let stand at room temperature for 30 minutes. The batter should be the consistency of heavy cream. If too thick, thin with a little water or milk. To make crepes, lightly coat an 8-inch nonstick skillet with flared sides with nonstick olive oil cooking spray. Preheat skillet over medium-low heat until a drop of water sizzles. Spoon in about ¼ cup of the batter; lift and tilt skillet to spread batter. Cook for 2 to 3 minutes or until browned on bottom and top looks dry. Carefully turn crepe; cook about 1 minute more or until the bottom is lightly browned but crepe is still pliable. Carefully invert onto waxed paper. Repeat with the remaining batter. Makes 8 crepes.

1. In a very large skillet heat the olive oil over medium-high heat. Add the mushrooms; cook for 8 to 10 minutes or until golden brown, stirring occasionally. Season to taste with kosher salt and pepper. Add the garlic; cook for 1 minute. Add the balsamic vinegar; cook and stir for 1 minute more. Add spinach, cheese, and basil; cook and stir for 1 to 2 minutes or until spinach is wilted.

2. Preheat broiler. Divide mushroom mixture among Basic Crepes or tortillas, using about ⅓ cup for each and spooning along the centers. Roll up crepes or tortillas. Place in a broilerproof 13×9×2-inch baking pan. Sprinkle with Parmesan cheese. Broil 3 to 4 inches from the heat for 1 to 2 minutes or just until the cheese starts to brown.

For Wave 1, serve with cooked broccoli or asparagus. For Waves 2 and 3, serve with fresh strawberries.

Wine Pairing: Pinot Noir

Olive Oil

Spinach

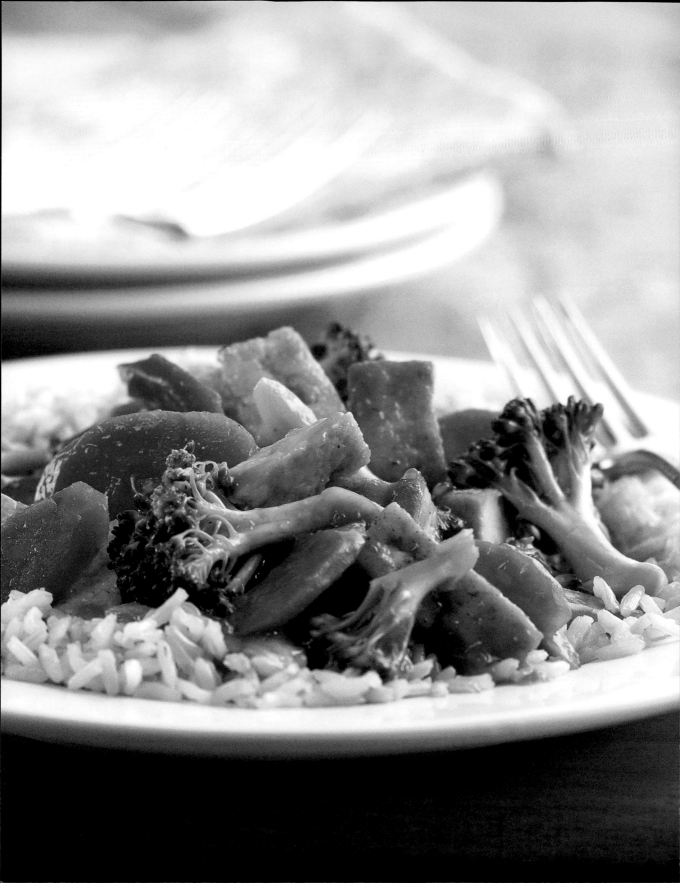

VEGETABLE AND TOFU STIR-FRY

SONOMA *express*

This nutritious stir-fry takes full advantage of tofu's health properties—high levels of isoflavones and protein, and zero cholesterol. Be sure all your prep work is complete before tossing ingredients into the wok; the stir-fry method requires constant, brisk stirring once the ingredients have been added.

Start to Finish: 30 minutes **Makes:** 4 servings

1½ cups instant brown rice

½ cup vegetable broth or chicken broth

¼ cup dry sherry

1 tablespoon cornstarch

1 tablespoon reduced-sodium soy sauce

1 teaspoon grated fresh ginger

½ teaspoon crushed red pepper (optional)

Nonstick olive oil cooking spray

1 cup thinly bias-sliced carrot

3 cloves garlic, minced (1½ teaspoons minced)

3 cups broccoli florets

6 ounces firm tofu (fresh bean curd), drained and cut into ½- to 1-inch cubes

1 cup fresh or frozen shelled green sweet soybeans (edamame), thawed if necessary (optional)

1. Prepare the rice according to package directions. Cover and keep warm.

2. For sauce, in a small bowl stir together broth, dry sherry, cornstarch, soy sauce, ginger, and, if desired, crushed red pepper. Set sauce aside.

3. Coat an unheated wok or large skillet with nonstick cooking spray. Preheat over medium-high heat. Add carrot and garlic to hot wok; stir-fry for 2 minutes. Add broccoli; stir-fry for 3 to 4 minutes more or until vegetables are crisp-tender. Push vegetables from center of wok.

4. Stir sauce; add to center of wok. Cook and stir until thickened and bubbly. Add tofu and, if desired, soybeans; gently stir together to coat all ingredients with sauce. Cook and stir gently for 1 minute more.

5. To serve, spoon vegetable mixture over hot cooked rice.

Nutrition facts per serving: 214 cal., 3 g total fat (0 g sat. fat), 0 mg chol., 315 mg sodium, 38 g carbo., 5 g fiber, 9 g pro.
Exchanges: 1 Vegetable, 2 Starch, ½ Lean Meat

For Wave 1, serve with a spinach salad. For Waves 2 and 3, serve with fresh kiwifruit.

Wine Pairing: sparkling semisweet

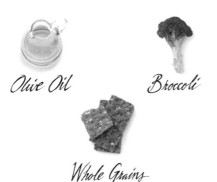

Olive Oil

Broccoli

Whole Grains

PAN-GRILLED MARINATED TOFU

Starting with firm tofu is important when marinating because, in order for the marinade to be absorbed, there has to be room for it. If the tofu is already filled with liquid, as with less-firm varieties, it cannot soak up the marinade.

Prep: 20 minutes **Cook:** 6 minutes **Marinate:** 30 minutes **Makes:** 4 servings

- 1   16-ounce package water-packed firm tofu (fresh bean curd), well drained
- 2   tablespoons chopped fresh stemmed shiitake mushrooms or 1 tablespoon dried shiitake or porcini mushrooms
- 2   tablespoons extra-virgin olive oil
- 2   tablespoons soy sauce
- 1   tablespoon red wine vinegar
- 1   tablespoon water
- 6   cloves garlic, minced (1 tablespoon minced)
- 1   tablespoon chopped fresh flat-leaf parsley
- ¼   teaspoon kosher salt
- ¼   teaspoon freshly ground black pepper

1. Cut tofu into 1-inch-thick slices. Arrange tofu slices in a 3-quart rectangular baking dish; set aside. If using dried mushrooms, in a small bowl combine dried mushrooms and enough hot water to cover; let stand for 5 minutes. Drain and rinse mushrooms; chop mushrooms.

2. For marinade, in a blender combine the mushrooms, 1 tablespoon of the olive oil, the soy sauce, vinegar, water, garlic, parsley, kosher salt, and pepper. Cover and blend until nearly smooth. Spoon mixture over tofu in dish. Turn tofu slices to coat with marinade. Cover and marinate at room temperature for 30 minutes, carefully turning tofu slices occasionally.

3. In a large skillet heat remaining 1 tablespoon olive oil over medium heat. Remove tofu slices from marinade, allowing excess to drip off; discard

marinade. Add tofu to skillet. Cook for 6 to 8 minutes or until browned and heated through, turning once.

Per serving: 239 cal., 17 g total fat (2 g sat. fat), 0 mg chol., 646 mg sodium, 8 g carbo., 3 g fiber, 19 g pro.
Exchanges: ½ Starch, 2½ Medium-Fat Meat, ½ Fat

Latin-Style Marinated Tofu: Prepare as directed, except add 2 to 3 canned chipotle peppers in adobo sauce and 1 teaspoon fresh oregano leaves to the blender with the other marinade ingredients.

Per serving: 240 cal., 17 g total fat (2 g sat. fat), 0 mg chol., 651 mg sodium, 8 g carbo., 3 g fiber, 19 g pro.
Exchanges: ½ Starch, 2½ Medium-Fat Meat, ½ Fat

Asian-Style Marinated Tofu: Prepare as directed, except substitute rice vinegar for the red wine vinegar and add 1 teaspoon grated fresh ginger and 1 teaspoon toasted sesame oil to the blender with the other marinade ingredients.

Nutrition facts per serving: 251 cal., 18 g total fat (3 g sat. fat), 0 mg chol., 646 mg sodium, 8 g carbo., 3 g fiber, 19 g pro.
Exchanges: ½ Starch, 2 ½ Medium-Fat Meat, ½ Fat

For Wave 1, serve with cooked brown rice and Roasted Green Beans (page 212). For Waves 2 and 3, serve with cooked brown rice, Roasted Green Beans (page 212), and fresh pineapple.

Wine Pairing: Chardonnay

Olive Oil

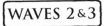
MEXICAN TOFU

This recipe transforms bland tofu into a full-flavored Mexican meal with only 30 minutes of marinating. When the tofu begins to form a light crust from grilling, you'll know it's done.

Prep: 20 minutes   **Marinate:** 30 minutes   **Grill:** 8 minutes   **Makes:** 4 servings

¼ cup lime juice

1 tablespoon extra-virgin olive oil

1 tablespoon chili powder or 2 teaspoons adobo sauce from canned chipotle chile peppers in adobo sauce

4 cloves garlic, minced (2 teaspoons minced)

¾ teaspoon ground cumin

1 16-ounce package refrigerated extra-firm water-packed tofu (fresh bean curd), well drained

1 cup fresh or frozen corn kernels

¾ teaspoon kosher salt

1 cup canned pinto beans, rinsed and drained

¾ cup bottled roasted red bell peppers, drained and chopped

½ cup pitted ripe olives, halved

2 tablespoons chopped fresh cilantro

2 tablespoons thinly sliced green onion

Olive Oil

Bell Peppers

1. In a shallow dish combine 2 tablespoons of the lime juice, 2 teaspoons of the olive oil, the chili powder or adobo sauce, garlic, and ¼ teaspoon of the cumin. Cut tofu into ½-inch-thick slices; add tofu slices to lime juice mixture, turning to coat. Cover and marinate in the refrigerator for 30 minutes.

2. Meanwhile, in a covered small saucepan cook corn in a small amount of boiling water for 3 minutes; drain well. Set aside. In a large bowl combine the remaining 2 tablespoons lime juice, the remaining 1 teaspoon olive oil, the remaining ½ teaspoon cumin, and ¼ teaspoon of the kosher salt. Add the drained corn, the beans, roasted bell peppers, olives, cilantro, and green onion. Set aside.

3. Remove tofu from marinade, reserving marinade. Sprinkle tofu with the remaining ½ teaspoon kosher salt. For a charcoal grill, place tofu on the greased rack of an uncovered grill directly over medium-hot coals. Grill for 8 to 10 minutes or until lightly browned and heated through, turning once and brushing occasionally with reserved marinade. (For a gas grill, preheat grill. Reduce heat to medium-high heat. Place tofu on greased grill rack over heat. Cover and grill as above.) Transfer tofu to four dinner plates; serve with corn mixture.

Nutrition facts per serving: 277 cal., 12 g total fat (2 g sat. fat), 0 mg chol., 710 mg sodium, 27 g carbo., 7 g fiber, 17 g pro.
Exchanges: ½ Vegetable, 1½ Starch, 2 Medium-Fat Meat

For Wave 1, this is not appropriate. For Waves 2 and 3, serve with fresh papaya.

Wine Pairing: sparkling semisweet

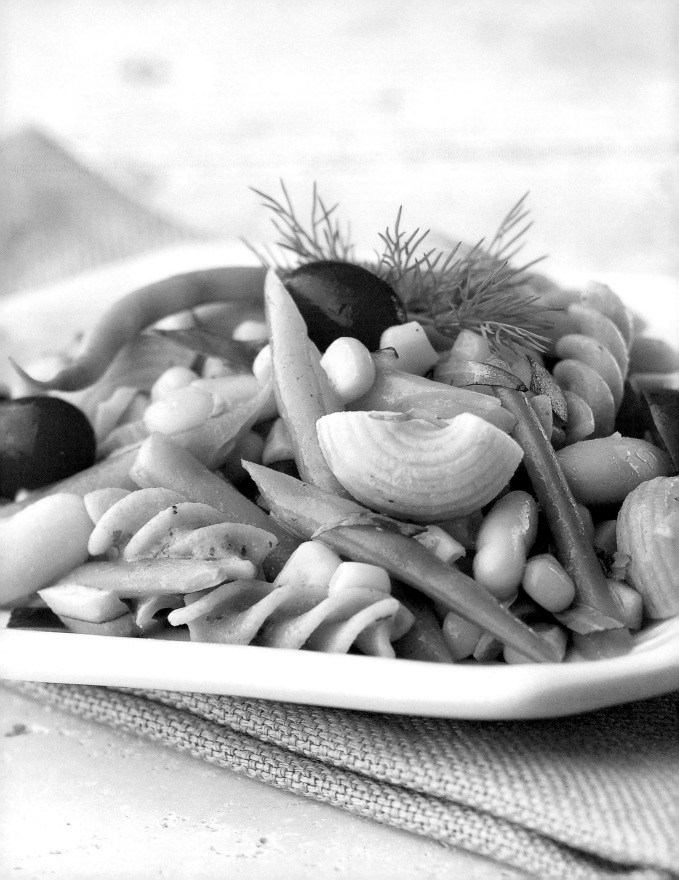

Side Dishes

Break out of the white rice or potatoes habit with these healthy, Sonoma Diet-friendly side dishes. How could a boiled potato stand up to Wine Country Grain Medley or roasted green beans? What's white rice compared to Basil Quinoa with Red Bell Pepper or Spicy Black-Eyed Pea Salad? Your plate deserves the best from edge to edge, and you'll find it here.

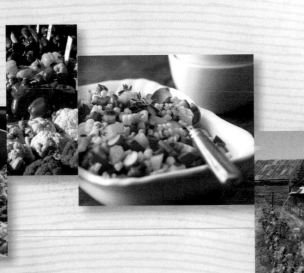

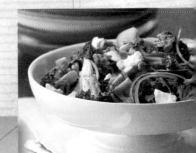

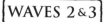

ROASTED RATATOUILLE

This popular French dish is loaded with Mediterranean veggies that have been roasted for intensified flavor. Ratatouille tastes great served warm or cold and pairs perfectly with almost any entree.

Prep: 15 minutes **Roast:** 20 minutes + 8 minutes **Oven:** 450°F **Makes:** 4 side-dish servings

Nonstick olive oil cooking spray

3½ cups cubed eggplant (1 small)

1 cup cubed yellow summer squash or zucchini (1 small)

8 pearl onions, halved

1 medium yellow bell pepper, cut into 1-inch strips

2 tablespoons chopped fresh flat-leaf parsley or regular parsley

1 tablespoon extra-virgin olive oil

2 cloves garlic, minced (1 teaspoon minced)

⅛ teaspoon kosher salt

⅛ teaspoon freshly ground black pepper

2 large tomatoes, chopped

1½ teaspoons lemon juice

1. Preheat oven to 450°F. Coat a 15×10×1-inch baking pan with nonstick cooking spray. Place eggplant, squash, onions, bell pepper, and parsley in the prepared pan.

2. In a small bowl stir together olive oil, garlic, kosher salt, and black pepper. Drizzle over vegetables; toss gently to coat. Spread in an even layer.

3. Roast about 20 minutes or until vegetables are tender and lightly brown, stirring once. Stir in the tomatoes and lemon juice. Roast, uncovered, for 8 to 10 minutes more or until tomatoes are very soft and starting to juice out.

Nutrition facts per serving: 87 cal., 4 g total fat (1 g sat. fat), 0 mg chol., 68 mg sodium, 13 g carbo., 4 g fiber, 2 g pro.
Exchanges: 2½ Vegetable, ½ Fat

Olive Oil

Tomatoes

Bell Peppers

WINTER SQUASH GRATIN

Mild mozzarella melts smoothly over tender, sweet squash slices to give this casserole a cheesy top layer. A tablespoon of fresh sage enhances the squash flavor for a grade-A gratin.

Prep. 30 minutes **Bake.** 45 minutes + 10 minutes **Stand:** 10 minutes **Oven:** 350°F **Makes:** 8 servings

Nonstick olive oil cooking spray

2 tablespoons extra-virgin olive oil

2 large onions, thinly sliced

6 cloves garlic, minced (1 tablespoon minced)

1 tablespoon chopped fresh sage

2 teaspoons chopped fresh thyme

¼ teaspoon kosher salt

¼ teaspoon freshly ground black pepper

2 pounds butternut squash, peeled, halved lengthwise, seeded, and cut crosswise into ¼-inch-thick slices

1½ cups soft whole wheat bread crumbs (about 2 slices)

1 tablespoon chopped fresh flat-leaf parsley

¾ cup shredded part-skim mozzarella cheese

¼ cup finely shredded Parmesan cheese (1 ounce)

1. Preheat oven to 350°F. Lightly coat a 2-quart square baking dish with nonstick cooking spray; set aside.

2. In a large skillet heat 1 tablespoon of the olive oil over medium heat. Add onions and garlic; cook about 6 minutes or until tender, stirring occasionally. Remove from heat. Stir in sage, thyme, kosher salt, and pepper.

3. Place half of the squash slices in the prepared dish. Sprinkle with the onion mixture and half of the bread crumbs. Top with remaining squash slices. Cover with foil. Bake about 45 minutes or until squash is nearly tender.

4. Meanwhile, in a small bowl combine the remaining bread crumbs, the remaining 1 tablespoon olive oil, and the parsley. Mix well and set aside.

5. Remove foil from baking dish; sprinkle squash with mozzarella cheese, Parmesan cheese, and bread crumb mixture. Bake, uncovered, for 10 to 15 minutes more or until crumbs are golden brown and squash is tender. Let stand for 10 minutes before serving.

Nutrition facts per serving: 150 cal., 6 g total fat (2 g sat. fat), 7 mg chol., 204 mg sodium, 21 g carbo., 3 g fiber, 5 g pro.
Exchanges: 1 Starch, ½ Lean Meat, 1 Fat

Olive Oil

Whole Grains

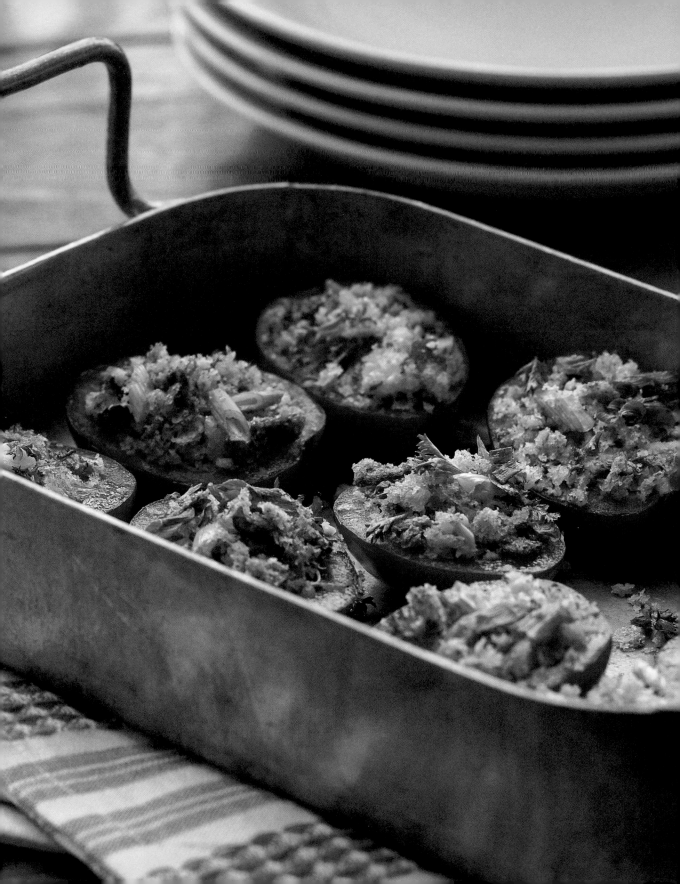

TOMATOES WITH CRISPY BREAD TOPPING

A basic herb of French cuisine, thyme is commonly used to add flavor to vegetables.
Here its small leaves contribute a strong, somewhat minty flavor to roasted tomatoes.

Prep: 20 minutes **Bake:** 15 minutes **Oven:** 400°F **Makes:** 4 servings

8   roma tomatoes, cored and cut in half lengthwise (about 1⅓ pounds)

   Kosher salt

   Freshly ground black pepper

½   cup soft whole wheat bread crumbs

¼   cup thinly sliced green onions

2   tablespoons chopped fresh thyme

1   tablespoon chopped fresh flat-leaf parsley

1   tablespoon chopped fresh tarragon

1   tablespoon extra-virgin olive oil

2   cloves garlic, minced (1 teaspoon minced)

1. Preheat oven to 400°F. Sprinkle the cut sides of the tomatoes with kosher salt and pepper. Arrange tomatoes, cut sides up, in a shallow baking pan. Set aside.

2. In a small bowl combine the bread crumbs, green onions, thyme, parsley, tarragon, olive oil, and garlic.° Sprinkle over tomato halves. Bake, uncovered, for 15 to 20 minutes or until the tomatoes are heated through and the bread crumbs are browned and crisp.

Nutrition facts per serving: 75 cal., 4 g total fat (1 g sat. fat), 0 mg chol., 152 mg sodium, 9 g carbo., 3 g fiber, 2 g pro.
Exchanges: 1½ Vegetable, 1 Fat

°**Note:** If desired, add 1 tablespoon grated Parmesan cheese to the bread crumb topping.

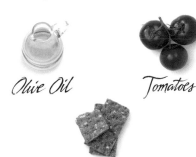

Olive Oil   *Tomatoes*

Whole Grains

CRUMB-TOPPED CAULIFLOWER

An excellent source of vitamin C, folate, fiber, and phytochemicals, cauliflower takes center stage in this side dish. The crumb topping adds a nice crunch and rich flavor to this versatile side dish

Prep: 25 minutes **Bake:** 15 minutes **Oven:** 375°F **Makes:** 6 servings

¼ cup extra-virgin olive oil

3 cloves garlic, minced (1½ teaspoons minced)

4 cups cauliflower florets

3 tablespoons lemon juice

2 tablespoons capers, rinsed and drained

2 tablespoons chopped fresh flat-leaf parsley

1 tablespoon finely chopped anchovy fillets (optional)

1 ounce thinly sliced prosciutto, cut into thin bite-size strips

Kosher salt

Freshly ground black pepper

1 cup soft whole wheat bread crumbs

1. Preheat oven to 375°F. In a large skillet heat 2 tablespoons of the olive oil over medium heat. Add garlic; cook and stir for 30 seconds. Add cauliflower; cook about 10 minutes or until tender, stirring frequently. Add lemon juice, capers, 1 tablespoon of the parsley, the anchovies (if desired), and prosciutto. Cook and stir for 2 minutes more. Season to taste with kosher salt and pepper.

2. Transfer cauliflower mixture to a 2-quart baking dish or au gratin dish. In a small bowl combine bread crumbs, the remaining 2 tablespoons olive oil, and the remaining 1 tablespoon parsley; sprinkle on top of cauliflower mixture.

3. Bake about 15 minutes or until crumbs are golden brown.

Nutrition facts per serving: 129 cal., 10 g total fat (1 g sat. fat), 0 mg chol., 298 mg sodium, 7 g carbo., 2 g fiber, 3 g pro.
Exchanges: 1 Vegetable, 2½ Fat

Olive Oil

Whole Grains

MUSHROOMS WITH GARLIC AND HERBS

Delicately flavored with garlic, thyme, and white wine, these mushrooms make an elegant, earthy side.

Start to Finish: 30 minutes **Makes:** 4 servings

1½ pounds assorted fresh mushrooms (such as button, cremini, porcini, chanterelle, and/or shiitake)

3 tablespoons extra-virgin olive oil

3 cloves garlic, thinly sliced

1 tablespoon chopped fresh thyme

¼ cup dry white wine

1 tablespoon lemon juice

Kosher salt

Freshly ground black pepper

2 tablespoons chopped fresh flat-leaf parsley

1. Trim off and discard mushroom stems. Leave mushrooms caps whole or thickly slice large caps.

2. In a very large skillet heat olive oil over medium-high heat. Add mushrooms; cook about 10 minutes or until lightly browned, stirring often.

3. Add the garlic and thyme; cook and stir for 1 minute. Add wine and lemon juice; cook for 1 minute more. Season to taste with kosher salt and pepper.

4. Transfer mushroom mixture to a serving dish. Sprinkle with parsley.

Nutrition facts per serving: 143 cal., 11 g total fat (1 g sat. fat), 0 mg chol., 130 mg sodium, 7 g carbo., 2 g fiber, 6 g pro.
Exchanges: 1½ Vegetable, 2½ Fat

Olive Oil

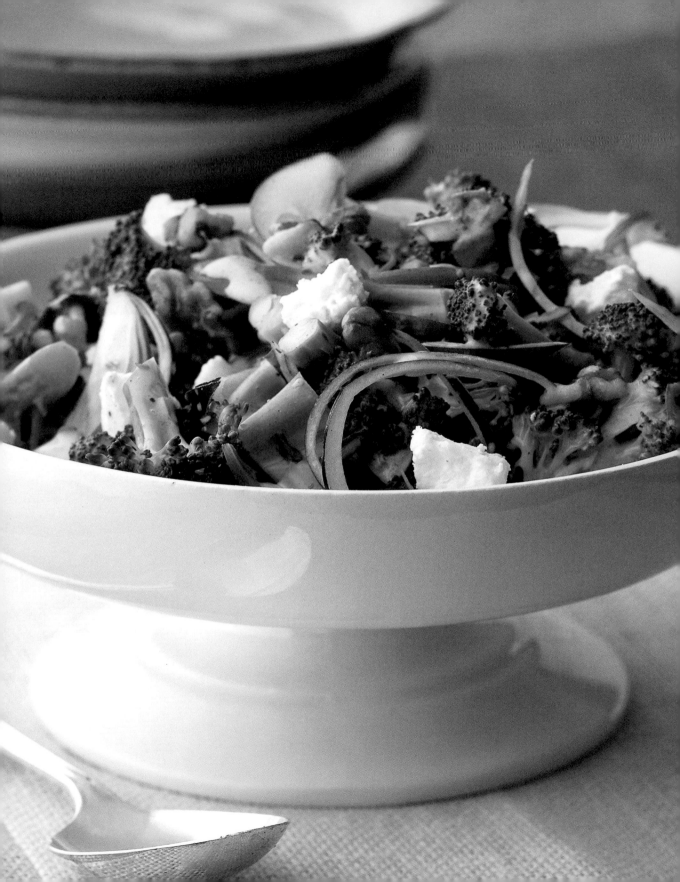

BROCCOLI WITH GOAT CHEESE AND WALNUTS

*Dressed up with tangy buttermilk and a topping of tart chèvre and walnuts,
this side dish runs the gamut of flavors. With broccoli as its star, this dish
is loaded with such nutrients as vitamins A and C and folate.*

Start to Finish: 30 minutes **Makes:** 6 servings

1 pound broccoli, trimmed and cut into 1-inch pieces

½ cup buttermilk

1 tablespoon chopped fresh flat-leaf parsley

1 tablespoon Dijon-style mustard

2 teaspoons extra-virgin olive oil

1 teaspoon chopped fresh thyme

1 teaspoon red wine vinegar

1 clove garlic, minced (½ teaspoon minced)

¼ teaspoon kosher salt

⅛ teaspoon ground nutmeg

⅛ teaspoon freshly ground black pepper

½ cup thinly slivered red onion

¼ cup coarsely chopped walnuts, toasted

1 ounce semisoft goat cheese (chèvre) or feta cheese, crumbled

1. In a covered large saucepan cook broccoli in a small amount of lightly salted boiling water for 6 to 8 minutes or until crisp-tender. Drain and set aside.

2. In a large bowl whisk together buttermilk, parsley, mustard, olive oil, thyme, red wine vinegar, garlic, kosher salt, nutmeg, and pepper. Add the broccoli and red onion; stir gently to coat. Top with walnuts and goat cheese.

Nutrition facts per serving: 105 cal., 7 g total fat (2 g sat. fat), 4 mg chol., 212 mg sodium, 9 g carbo., 3 g fiber, 5 g pro.
Exchanges: 1½ Vegetable, 1½ Fat

Make-ahead directions: Prepare as directed, except do not top with walnuts and goat cheese. Cover and chill for up to 4 hours. To serve, top with walnuts and goat cheese.

Olive Oil

Broccoli

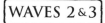
ROASTED GREEN BEANS

*There's nothing to these roasted beans–simply trim the stems and ends, toss with oil, and roast.
There are several variations to try, and if you're not a fan of green beans,
you can use asparagus as a delicious alternative.*

Prep: 15 minutes **Roast:** 10 minutes + 10 minutes **Oven:** 450°F **Makes:** 6 servings

1 pound fresh green beans, trimmed*
1 tablespoon extra-virgin olive oil
   Kosher salt
   Freshly ground black pepper

1. Preheat oven to 450°F. Line a baking sheet with foil. Place beans on prepared baking sheet.

2. Drizzle the beans with olive oil and sprinkle with kosher salt and black pepper; toss gently to coat. Spread the beans in an even layer. Roast for 10 minutes.

3. Stir beans. Roast about 10 minutes more or until beans are dark golden brown in spots and have started to shrivel.

Per serving: 43 cal., 2 g total fat (0 g sat. fat), 0 mg chol., 85 mg sodium, 5 g carbo., 3 g fiber, 1 g pro.
Exchanges: 1 Vegetable, ½ Fat

Roasted Green Beans with Red Onion and Walnuts: Prepare as directed through step 2, except add ½ of a medium red onion, cut into ½-inch-thick wedges, to the beans before roasting. Meanwhile, in a small bowl combine 1 tablespoon balsamic vinegar, 1 teaspoon chopped fresh thyme, 1 teaspoon honey, and 2 cloves garlic, minced (1 teaspoon minced). Drizzle vinegar mixture over green bean mixture; toss gently to coat. Spread in an even layer. Roast about 10 minutes more or until beans are dark golden brown in spots and have started to shrivel. To serve, sprinkle with ⅓ cup chopped walnuts, toasted.

Nutrition facts per serving: 97 cal., 7 g total fat (1 g sat. fat), 0 mg chol., 86 mg sodium, 9 g carbo., 3 g fiber, 3 g pro.
Exchanges: 1 Vegetable, 1 ½ Fat

Roasted Sesame-Ginger Green Beans: Prepare as directed through step 2. Meanwhile, in a small bowl combine 1 tablespoon soy sauce; 6 cloves garlic, minced (1 tablespoon minced); 2 teaspoons honey; 1 teaspoon grated fresh ginger; ½ teaspoon toasted sesame oil; and ¼ teaspoon crushed red pepper. Drizzle soy sauce mixture over green beans; toss gently to coat. Spread in an even layer. Roast about 10 minutes more or until beans are dark golden brown in spots and have started to shrivel. To serve, sprinkle with 4 teaspoons sesame seeds, toasted.

Nutrition facts per serving: 72 cal., 4 g total fat (1 g sat. fat), 0 mg chol., 255 mg sodium, 9 g carbo., 3 g fiber, 2 g pro.
Exchanges: 1 Vegetable, 1 Fat

Roasted Green Beans with Dried Tomatoes, Goat Cheese, and Olives: Prepare as directed through step 3. Meanwhile, in a large bowl combine ¼ cup coarsely chopped drained oil-packed dried tomatoes; ¼ cup pitted kalamata olives, quartered lengthwise, or sliced pitted ripe olives; 1 tablespoon chopped fresh oregano; and 1 tablespoon lemon juice. Add roasted green beans; toss gently to coat. To serve, sprinkle with ½ cup crumbled goat cheese or feta cheese.

Nutrition facts per serving: 98 cal., 7 g total fat (2 g sat. fat), 7 mg chol., 208 mg sodium, 8 g carbo., 3 g fiber, 4 g pro.
Exchanges: 1 Vegetable, 1 ½ Fat

*Note: This recipe is delicious with asparagus in place of green beans. Just reduce the roasting time to 15 minutes total.

Olive Oil

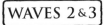
ARTICHOKE SALAD

Artichokes are low in calories but dense in an assortment of beneficial nutrients.
If you're new to cooking baby artichokes, here's a tip: They're done
when the bottoms can be pierced with the tip of a knife.

Prep: 30 minutes **Chill:** 2 to 4 hours **Makes:** 6 side-dish servings

10 baby artichokes or two 8-ounce packages frozen artichoke hearts or two 14-ounce cans artichoke hearts

2 tablespoons lemon juice

2 tablespoons chopped fresh mint

1 teaspoon finely shredded lemon peel

2 tablespoons lemon juice

4 teaspoons extra-virgin olive oil

¼ teaspoon kosher salt

⅛ teaspoon freshly ground black pepper

2 cloves garlic, minced (1 teaspoon minced)

1 small bulb fennel, halved and cored

½ of a small red onion

1 cup halved cherry tomatoes

Olive Oil

Tomatoes

1. To prepare baby artichokes, trim stems; cut off top one-fourth of each artichoke. Remove outer leaves until you reach the pale green parts. Halve or cut artichokes into wedges. Brush cut edges with some of the 2 tablespoons lemon juice; add remaining lemon juice to cooking water. In a large saucepan cook artichokes in a large amount of boiling water for 12 to 15 minutes or until tender; drain. (Or cook frozen artichoke hearts according to package directions; drain.) Rinse artichokes with cold water. Drain and place in a large bowl.

2. Meanwhile, for dressing, in a small bowl combine mint, lemon peel, lemon juice, olive oil, kosher salt, pepper, and garlic.

3. Thinly slice fennel and red onion. Add fennel, red onion, and tomatoes to artichokes. Pour dressing over; toss to coat.

4. Cover and chill for 2 to 4 hours. Serve chilled or at room temperature.

Nutrition facts per serving: 82 cal., 4 g total fat (0 g sat. fat), 0 mg chol., 143 mg sodium, 11 g carbo., 6 g fiber, 3 g pro.
Exchanges: 2 Vegetable, ½ Fat

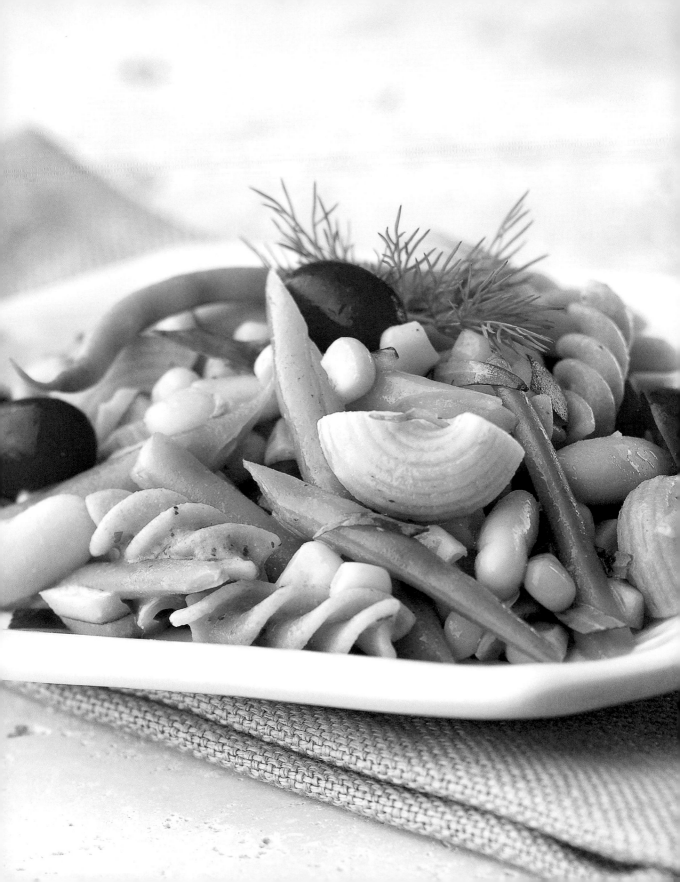

CORN, BEAN, AND TOMATO SALAD

This stunning side salad has it all! Red tomatoes, yellow corn, and green beans make a colorful mosaic for your plate and can be served at room temperature or chilled.

Start to Finish: 25 minutes **Makes:** 4 servings

½ cup dried multigrain rotini, elbow macaroni, and/or penne pasta (such as Barilla Plus)

8 ounces fresh green beans or frozen whole green beans, halved if desired

1 cup frozen whole kernel corn, thawed

1 cup cherry tomatoes, halved

½ cup canned cannellini beans (white kidney beans), rinsed and drained

2 tablespoons white wine vinegar

2 tablespoons extra-virgin olive oil

2 tablespoons finely chopped red onion

1 tablespoon Dijon-style mustard

1 tablespoon chopped fresh tarragon

Fresh dill (optional)

1. In a large saucepan bring 2 quarts of lightly salted water to boiling. Add pasta and, if using, fresh beans. Cook according to pasta package directions, adding frozen green beans (if using) for the last 5 minutes of cooking. Drain pasta and beans.

2. In a large bowl combine the pasta, green beans, corn, tomatoes, and cannellini beans; set aside. For dressing, in a small bowl whisk together the vinegar, olive oil, red onion, mustard, and tarragon until well mixed. Pour dressing over vegetable mixture; toss well to combine. If desired, garnish with fresh dill.

Nutrition facts per serving: 192 cal., 8 g total fat (1 g sat. fat), 0 mg chol., 157 mg sodium, 28 g carbo., 6 g fiber, 8 g pro.
Exchanges: 1 Vegetable, 1 Starch, 1½ Fat

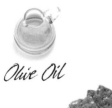

Olive Oil

Tomatoes

Whole Grains

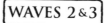 # SPICY BLACK-EYED PEA SALAD

Featuring black-eyed peas, a staple of Southern cooking, this chunky salad gets its spicy taste from serrano chile pepper. A range is given for this ingredient so you can choose the level of spiciness.

Start to Finish: 25 minutes **Makes:** 8 servings

2   15-ounce cans black-eyed peas, rinsed and drained

2   cups frozen whole kernel corn, thawed, or one 15¼-ounce can whole kernel corn, drained

2   cups chopped, seeded cucumber

2   cups chopped, seeded tomato

½   cup chopped red onion

¼   cup chopped fresh cilantro

3   tablespoons lemon juice

1   tablespoon extra-virgin olive oil

2   to 3 teaspoons finely chopped fresh serrano chile pepper*

¾   teaspoon kosher salt

½   teaspoon freshly ground black pepper

1. In a large bowl combine black-eyed peas, corn, cucumber, tomato, red onion, cilantro, lemon juice, olive oil, chile pepper, kosher salt, and black pepper. Gently stir to combine.

Nutrition facts per serving: 170 cal., 3 g total fat (0 g sat. fat), 0 mg chol., 483 mg sodium, 30 g carbo., 7 g fiber, 8 g pro.
Exchanges: 1 Vegetable, 1½ Starch, ½ Fat

Make-ahead directions: Prepare as directed. Cover and chill for up to 24 hours.

*See note, page 76

Olive Oil

Tomatoes

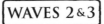

BROWN RICE PILAF

This warm and creamy side dish will boost the percentages of vegetables and protein on your plate.
Brown rice also boosts the manganese, selenium, and tryptophan content of your meal.

Prep: 20 minutes **Cook:** 45 minutes **Stand:** 10 minutes **Makes:** 8 side-dish servings

1   tablespoon extra-virgin olive oil

1   cup chopped onion

1   cup chopped celery

1   cup chopped carrot

3   cloves garlic, minced (1½ teaspoons minced)

2   teaspoons chopped fresh thyme

¼   teaspoon kosher salt

¼   teaspoon freshly ground black pepper

1   cup long grain brown rice or red rice*

2¼ cups vegetable stock or vegetable broth

1   tablespoon chopped fresh flat-leaf parsley

    Kosher salt (optional)

    Freshly ground black pepper (optional)

1. In a large saucepan heat olive oil over medium heat. Add the onion, celery, and carrot. Cook and stir about 4 minutes or until tender. Add garlic, thyme, the ¼ teaspoon salt, and the ¼ teaspoon pepper. Cook and stir for 1 minute. Add the uncooked rice; stir to combine.

2. Add the stock or broth. Bring to boiling; reduce heat. Cover and simmer about 45 minutes or until the rice is tender.

3. Remove from heat; let stand, covered, for 10 minutes. Fluff gently with a fork; stir in parsley. If desired, season to taste with additional kosher salt and pepper.

Nutrition facts per serving: 124 cal., 2 g total fat
(0 g sat. fat), 0 mg chol., 350 mg sodium, 23 g carbo.,
2 g fiber, 2 g pro.
Exchanges: ½ Vegetable, 1 Starch, ½ Fat

*Note: If using red rice, decrease vegetable broth to 2 cups and simmer for 30 minutes in step 2.

Olive Oil

Whole Grains

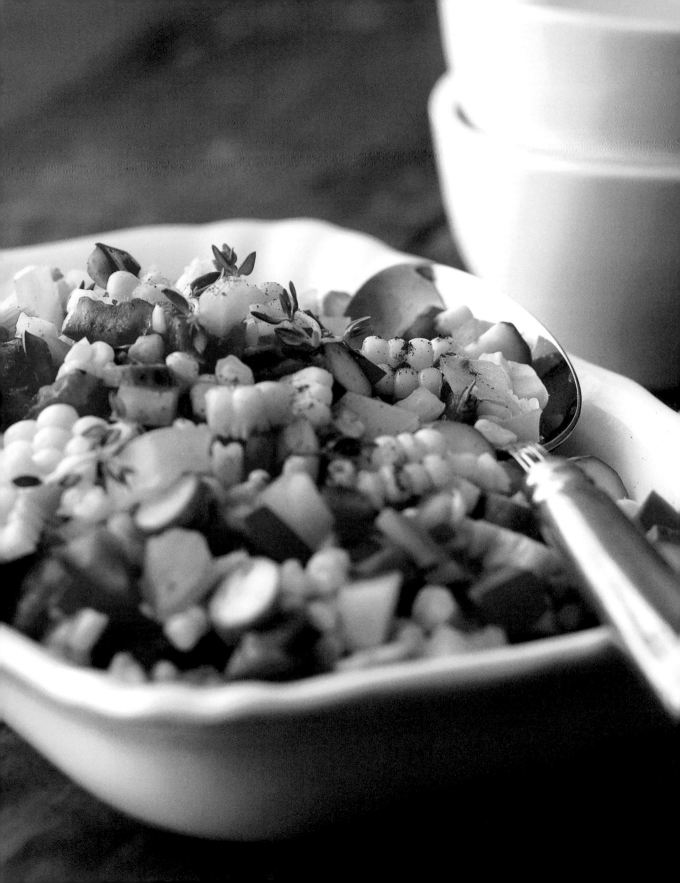

CONFETTI SUMMER SALAD

*Fresh, crisp, and colorful is just what you're looking for in a summer salad.
The fresh veggies in this dish are most abundant during summer months
but are available yearlong, so the salad never goes out of season.*

Prep: 30 minutes **Chill:** 4 to 24 hours **Makes:** 8 side-dish servings

4 medium ears fresh corn or 2 cups frozen whole kernel corn, thawed

4 baby zucchini, thinly sliced, or ½ of a small zucchini, halved lengthwise and thinly sliced (½ cup)

2 medium tomatoes, seeded and chopped

2 green onions, sliced

1 medium yellow bell pepper, seeded and chopped

1 medium red bell pepper, seeded and chopped

½ cup bottled clear Italian salad dressing (such as Newman's Own brand)

¼ teaspoon cayenne pepper (optional)

Fresh thyme (optional)

1. If using fresh corn, in a covered large saucepan cook ears of corn in a small amount of boiling water for 4 minutes. Drain; rinse with cold water to cool. When cool enough to handle, cut corn from cobs (you should have about 2 cups corn kernels).

2. In a large bowl combine fresh cooked corn or thawed corn, zucchini, tomatoes, green onions, bell peppers, salad dressing, and, if desired, cayenne pepper. Cover and chill for 4 to 24 hours, stirring occasionally. If desired, garnish with fresh thyme.

Nutrition facts per serving: 99 cal., 5 g total fat (1 g sat. fat), 0 mg chol., 253 mg sodium, 14 g carbo., 2 g fiber, 2 g pro.
Exchanges: 1 Vegetable, ½ Starch, 1 Fat

Bell Peppers

Tomatoes

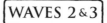

WINE COUNTRY GRAIN MEDLEY

*The Napa Valley and Sonoma regions are known for their rustic elegance;
you'll find these same elements in this recipe. The rustic feel comes from the
quinoa grain, sun-ripened tomatoes, and zucchini, which offer simple elegance.*

Prep: 10 minutes **Cook:** 15 minutes **Stand:** 5 minutes **Makes:** 6 servings

1   tablespoon extra-virgin olive oil

1   cup quartered fresh mushrooms

1½ cups water

¾   cup quinoa*

1   cup canned red beans, rinsed and drained

1   cup chopped zucchini

1   cup cherry tomatoes, halved if desired

1   tablespoon chopped fresh basil

1   tablespoon red wine vinegar

6   cloves garlic, minced (1 tablespoon minced)

¼   teaspoon kosher salt

¼   teaspoon freshly ground black pepper

1. In a very large skillet heat olive oil over medium heat. Add mushrooms; cook about 5 minutes or until golden brown, stirring occasionally. Add the water; bring to boiling. Add quinoa. Return to boiling; reduce heat. Cover and simmer about 15 minutes or until liquid is nearly absorbed. Stir in beans, zucchini, tomatoes, basil, vinegar, garlic, kosher salt, and pepper. Heat through. Remove from heat; let stand, covered, for 5 minutes before serving.

Nutrition facts per serving: 148 cal., 4 g total fat (0 g sat. fat), 0 mg chol., 247 mg sodium, 24 g carbo., 4 g fiber, 6 g pro.
Exchanges: ½ Vegetable, 1½ Starch, ½ Fat

*Note: Look for quinoa at a health food store or in the grains section of a large supermarket.

Olive Oil

Tomatoes

Whole Grains

BASIL QUINOA WITH RED BELL PEPPER

With quinoa playing the starring role, nutrients abound in this full-flavored grain side dish.
A great addition to any dinner, this dish goes especially well with a crisp salad.

Start to Finish: 25 minutes **Makes:** 8 servings

1 cup lightly packed fresh basil leaves

2 tablespoons freshly grated
    Parmesan cheese

2 tablespoons lemon juice

2 tablespoons extra-virgin olive oil

4 cloves garlic, minced (2 teaspoons
    minced)

2 cups cooked quinoa*

1 cup chopped red bell pepper

½ cup sliced green onions

    Kosher salt

    Freshly ground black pepper

¼ cup shelled sunflower seeds

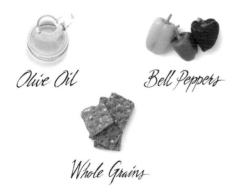

Olive Oil

Bell Peppers

Whole Grains

1. In a small saucepan bring 2 cups water to boiling. In a small bowl combine cold water and ice cubes to make an ice bath. Add the basil to the boiling water; stir once and drain immediately. Place basil in the ice bath to cool quickly. Gently squeeze out any excess water.

2. Place basil in a food processor. Add Parmesan cheese, lemon juice, olive oil, and garlic. Cover and process until nearly smooth.

3. In a medium bowl stir together cooked quinoa, bell pepper, and green onions. Add basil mixture; stir to coat. Season to taste with kosher salt and black pepper. Sprinkle with sunflower seeds.

Nutrition facts per serving: 123 cal., 7 g total fat (1 g sat. fat), 1 mg chol., 115 mg sodium, 13 g carbo., 2 g fiber, 4 g pro.
Exchanges: 1 Starch, 1 Fat

Make-ahead directions: Prepare as directed, except do not sprinkle with sunflower seeds. Cover and chill for up to 6 hours. To serve, sprinkle with sunflower seeds.

*Note: Look for quinoa at a health food store or in the grains section of a large supermarket. To make 2 cups cooked quinoa, in a fine strainer rinse ⅔ cup quinoa under cold running water; drain. In a small saucepan combine 1⅓ cups water, the quinoa, and ¼ teaspoon kosher salt. Bring to boiling; reduce heat. Cover and simmer for 15 minutes. Let stand to cool slightly. Drain off any remaining liquid.

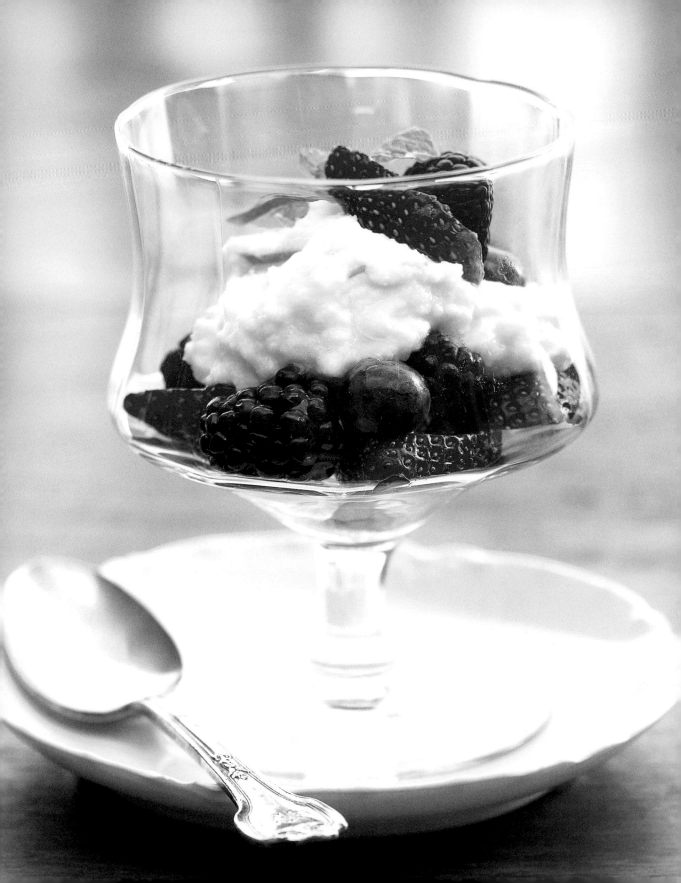

Snacks & Desserts

The Sonoma Diet encourages light between-meal snacking to calm your appetite and an occasional healthy indulgence after a meal. The challenge is snacking without chips or processed flour products and having dessert without excessive amounts of sugar. Here are solutions for you. For example, instead of ice cream, try a Ricotta Mousse with Berries. Instead of potato chips, go for Spiced-Roasted Almonds.

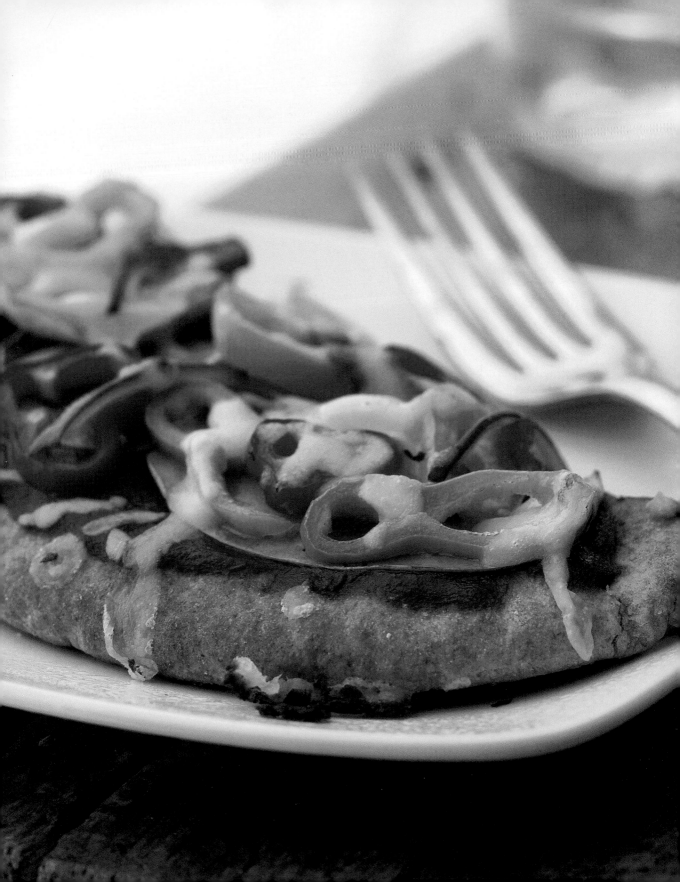

VEGETABLE PITA PIZZAS

Choose your favorite Wave-appropriate veggies and start piling them on! Check the labels on different pizza sauces and pick the one with the lowest amount of sugar.

Prep: 10 minutes **Bake:** 5 minutes + 8 minutes **Oven:** 400°F **Makes:** 4 servings

2 large whole wheat pita bread rounds

Nonstick olive oil cooking spray

1 cup assorted fresh vegetables (such as small broccoli or cauliflower florets, red bell pepper strips, sliced fresh mushrooms, and/or chopped carrot)

¼ cup pizza sauce

1 tablespoon chopped fresh herbs, such as basil, oregano, flat-leaf parsley, and/or thyme

½ cup spinach leaves

¼ cup shredded mozzarella cheese (1 ounce)

1. Preheat oven to 400°F. Place pita bread rounds on a baking sheet. Bake for 5 minutes.

2. Meanwhile, coat an unheated large skillet with nonstick cooking spray. Preheat over medium heat. Add the vegetables; cook and stir until crisp-tender.

3. In a small bowl combine pizza sauce and herbs. Spread on pita bread rounds; top with spinach leaves. Top with cooked vegetables and cheese. Bake for 8 to 10 minutes more or until lightly browned. Serve warm.

Nutrition facts per serving: 120 cal., 2 g total fat (1 g sat. fat), 4 mg chol., 303 mg sodium, 21 g carbo., 3 g fiber, 6 g pro.
Exchanges: ½ Vegetable, 1 Starch, ½ Fat

Bell Peppers

Whole Grains

Broccoli

Tomatoes

Spinach

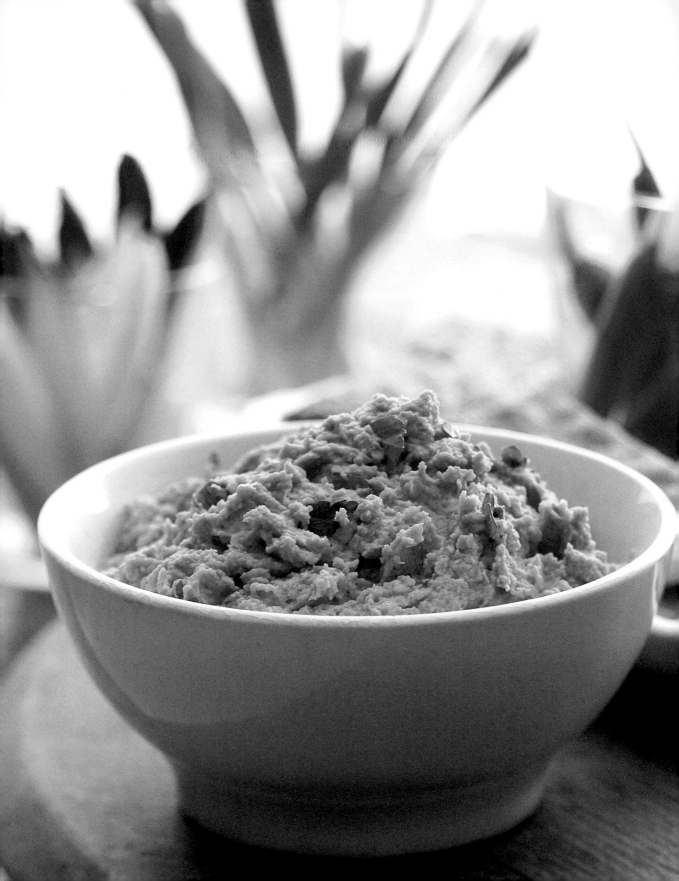

CARROT HUMMUS

Made of ground sesame seeds, tahini is commonly found in dishes of the Middle East, such as hummus. The addition of chopped carrots gives this hummus intensified color and sweetness.

Prep: 15 minutes **Chill:** 1 hour to 3 days **Makes:** 2 cups

1 cup chopped carrots

1 15-ounce can garbanzo beans (chickpeas), rinsed and drained

¼ cup tahini (sesame seed paste)

2 tablespoons lemon juice

2 cloves garlic, quartered

½ teaspoon ground cumin

¼ teaspoon kosher salt

2 tablespoons chopped fresh flat-leaf parsley

Assorted dippers (such as toasted whole wheat pita bread triangles, fresh vegetable dippers, and/or whole-grain crackers)

1. In a covered small saucepan cook carrots in a small amount of boiling water for 6 to 8 minutes or until tender; drain. In a food processor combine cooked carrots, garbanzo beans, tahini, lemon juice, garlic, cumin, and kosher salt. Cover and process until smooth. Transfer to a small serving bowl. Stir in 1 tablespoon of the parsley. Sprinkle top with remaining parsley.

2. Cover and chill for 1 hour to 3 days. If necessary, stir in enough water, 1 tablespoon at a time, to make dipping consistency. Serve with assorted dippers.

Nutrition facts per 2-tablespoon serving hummus: 58 cal., 2 g total fat (0 g sat. fat), 0 mg chol., 117 mg sodium, 8 g carbo., 2 g fiber, 2 g pro. Exchanges: ½ Starch, ½ Fat

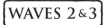
ROASTED EGGPLANT AND CAPER DIP

It may look like a lot of work, but once you've made this dip,
you can refrigerate and snack on it for up to a week with no fuss.

Prep: 30 minutes **Roast:** 40 minutes **Cool:** 30 minutes **Oven:** 400°F/425°F **Makes:** 4 cups

2   medium eggplant (about 2 pounds total)

1   cup chopped sweet onion (such as Vidalia, Walla Walla, or Maui)

1   tablespoon extra-virgin olive oil

6   cloves garlic, minced (1 tablespoon minced)

1   tablespoon chopped fresh oregano

2   tablespoons lemon juice

1/8 to 1/4 teaspoon cayenne pepper

1   cup bottled roasted red bell peppers, chopped

1/4 cup capers, rinsed, drained, and chopped

1   tablespoon chopped fresh flat-leaf parsley

1/2 teaspoon kosher salt

1/4 teaspoon freshly ground black pepper

8   large whole wheat pita bread rounds, cut into wedges and toasted*

Olive Oil

Bell Peppers

Whole Grains

1. Preheat oven to 400°F. Use a fork to pierce the skin of the eggplant all over. Place eggplant in a 15×10×1-inch baking pan. Roast about 40 minutes or until tender. Wrap eggplant tightly in foil. Cool about 30 minutes or until cool enough to handle. Remove the skin and discard; cut eggplant flesh into several large pieces.

2. Meanwhile, in a large skillet cook onion in hot olive oil about 7 minutes or until tender, stirring occasionally. Stir in garlic and oregano; cook about 3 minutes more or until fragrant, stirring occasionally.

3. In a food processor combine eggplant pieces, onion mixture, lemon juice, and cayenne pepper. Cover and pulse with several on/off turns until eggplant is coarsely chopped. Transfer to a large bowl. Stir in roasted bell peppers, capers, parsley, kosher salt, and black pepper. Serve with pita wedges.

Nutrition facts per 2-tablespoon serving with 4 pita wedges: 58 cal., 1 g total fat (0 g sat. fat), 0 mg chol., 148 mg sodium, 12 g carbo., 2 g fiber, 2 g pro. Exchanges: 1/2 Vegetable, 1/2 Starch

Make-ahead directions: Prepare dip as directed. Cover and chill for up to 1 week. Serve with pita wedges.

*Note: Preheat oven to 425°F. Cut pita bread rounds into 8 wedges each; split each wedge in half horizontally. Place wedges on ungreased baking sheets in a single layer. Bake about 7 minutes or until lightly browned and crisp. Cool on a wire rack. Makes 128 wedges.

WHITE BEAN AND ARTICHOKE DIP

Artichokes are naturally fat free and are a good source of fiber, vitamin C, and folate.
Enjoy their delicate flavor and nutritional benefits in this smooth, creamy dip.

Prep: 30 minutes **Bake:** 10 minutes per batch (pita chips) **Chill:** 2 to 24 hours **Oven:** 350°F **Makes:** 10 servings

2 tablespoons extra-virgin olive oil

12 cloves garlic, thinly sliced

1 cup chopped onion

1 tablespoon chopped fresh thyme

1 19-ounce can cannellini beans (white kidney beans), rinsed and drained

1 14-ounce can artichoke hearts, rinsed and drained

1 tablespoon lemon juice

⅛ teaspoon cayenne pepper

1 recipe Whole Wheat Pita Chips or 8 cups assorted vegetable dippers (such as carrot sticks, celery sticks, and/or red bell pepper strips)

Olive Oil

Whole Grains

1. In a large skillet heat olive oil over medium heat. Add thinly sliced garlic; cook for 5 to 7 minutes or until garlic is tender and golden brown (reduce heat to medium-low if garlic is browning too quickly). Stir in onion and thyme. Cook and stir about 5 minutes more or until onion is tender.

2. In a food processor combine cooked onion mixture, cannellini beans, artichoke hearts, lemon juice, and cayenne pepper. Cover and process until smooth. Cover and chill for 2 to 24 hours.

3. Serve with Whole Wheat Pita Chips or vegetable dippers.

Nutrition facts per 2 tablespoons dip and 3 pita wedges: 91 cal., 2 g total fat (0 g sat. fat), 0 mg chol., 220 mg sodium, 16 g carbo., 4 g fiber, 4 g pro. Exchanges: 1 Starch, ½ Fat

Whole Wheat Pita Chips: Preheat oven to 350°F. Split 4 large whole wheat pita bread rounds in half horizontally. Cut each half into six wedges. Arrange pita wedges in a single layer on an ungreased baking sheet. Bake for 10 to 12 minutes or until wedges are browned and crisp. (Bake the wedges in batches.) Store in an airtight container at room temperature for up to 1 week. Makes 48 chips.

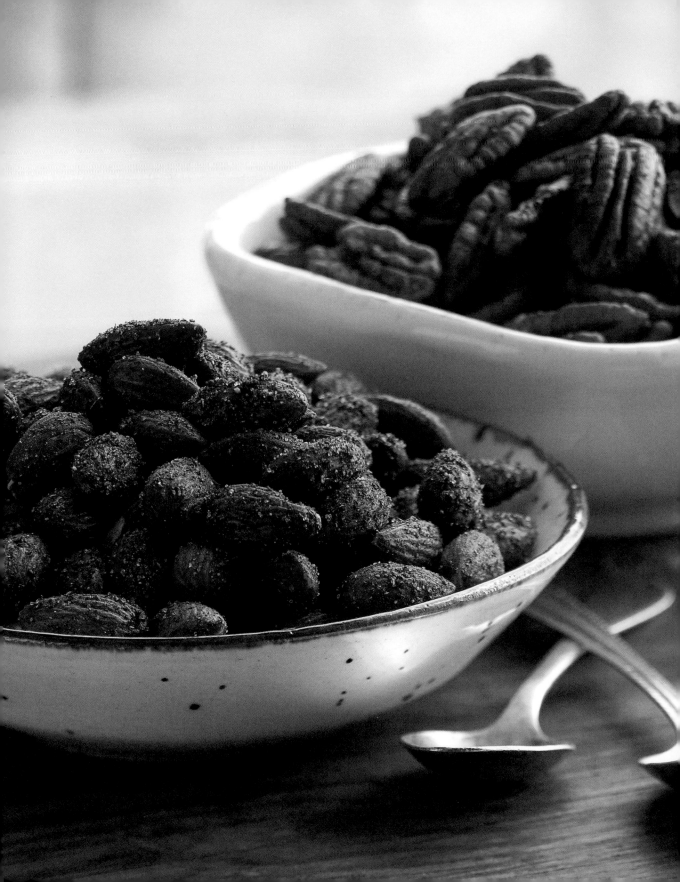

SPICE-ROASTED ALMONDS

This savory snack showcases the top Sonoma Power Food. These almonds are given a treatment of spices and a short baking time for amazing rich flavor and intense crunch.

Prep: 10 minutes **Bake:** 10 minutes **Oven:** 350°F **Makes:** 32 (1-tablespoon) servings

1 tablespoon chili powder	**1.** Preheat oven to 350°F. In a medium bowl combine chili powder, olive oil, kosher salt, cumin, coriander, cinnamon, and pepper; add almonds and toss to coat. Transfer mixture to a 13×9×2-inch baking pan.
1 tablespoon extra-virgin olive oil	
½ teaspoon kosher salt	
½ teaspoon ground cumin	
½ teaspoon ground coriander	**2.** Bake about 10 minutes or until almonds are toasted, stirring twice. Cool almonds completely before serving. Store in an airtight container for up to 5 days.
¼ teaspoon ground cinnamon	
¼ teaspoon freshly ground black pepper	
2 cups whole almonds	

Nutrition facts per serving: 62 cal., 5 g total fat (0 g sat. fat), 0 mg chol., 33 mg sodium, 2 g carbo., 1 g fiber, 2 g pro.
Exchanges: 1 Fat

Olive Oil

Almonds

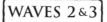 # SOY-GINGER ROASTED NUTS

Not all fats are created equal. Although this snack has higher fat content, it is primarily polyunsaturated fats from the pecans. Pecans are cholesterol free and a good source of omega-3 fatty acids, fiber, iron, and ellagic acid, which has been found to have anticancer properties. Pictured on page 230.

Prep: 5 minutes **Bake:** 10 minutes **Oven:** 350°F **Makes:** 2 cups

2 cups pecan halves

2 tablespoons reduced-sodium soy sauce

1 teaspoon toasted sesame oil

½ teaspoon ground ginger

⅛ to ¼ teaspoon cayenne pepper

1. Preheat oven to 350°F. Line a 15×10×1-inch baking pan with foil; set aside.

2. In a medium bowl combine pecans, soy sauce, sesame oil, ginger, and cayenne pepper. Spread pecan mixture in a single layer in prepared baking pan. Bake for 10 minutes, stirring once. Spread pecans on a sheet of foil; cool completely. Store in an airtight container for up to 2 weeks.

Nutrition facts per 2-tablespoon serving: 97 cal., 10 g total fat (1 g sat. fat), 0 mg chol., 72 mg sodium, 2 g carbo., 1 g fiber, 1 g pro.
Exchanges: 2 Fat

MOZZARELLA WITH HERBS

Hailing from Italy, mild-flavor mozzarella is perfectly complemented by this assortment of herbs and spices.

Prep: 15 minutes **Stand:** 30 minutes **Chill:** 2 to 4 hours **Makes:** 8 servings

8 ounces part-skim mozzarella cheese, cut into bite-size pieces (2 cups)

2 tablespoons extra-virgin olive oil

2 tablespoons chopped fresh basil

1 tablespoon chopped fresh oregano

1 tablespoon chopped fresh flat-leaf parsley

Kosher salt

Freshly ground black pepper

Olive Oil

1. In a medium bowl combine mozzarella cheese, olive oil, basil, oregano, and parsley. Cover and chill for 2 to 4 hours.

2. Let stand at room temperature for 30 minutes before serving. Season to taste with kosher salt and pepper.

Nutrition facts per serving: 103 cal., 8 g total fat (3 g sat. fat), 18 mg chol., 206 mg sodium, 1 g carbo., 0 g fiber, 7 g pro.
Exchanges: 1 Lean Meat, 1 Fat

Tomato-Mozzarella Salad: Prepare as directed, except add 4 cups roma tomato wedges and 2 tablespoons balsamic vinegar. Serve on a bed of 6 cups fresh spinach. Makes 6 servings.

Nutrition facts per serving: 169 cal., 11 g fat (5 g sat. fat), 24 mg chol., 304 mg sodium, 8 g carbo., 2 g fiber, 11 g pro.
Exchanges: 1½ Vegetable, 1½ Lean Meat, 1 Fat

Spicy Monterey Jack Cheese with Herbs: Prepare as directed, except substitute reduced-fat Monterey Jack cheese for the mozzarella cheese and add ½ teaspoon crushed red pepper. Makes 8 servings.

Nutrition facts per serving: 111 cal., 9 g fat (4 g sat. fat), 20 mg chol., 271 mg sodium, 1 g carbo., 0 g fiber, 7 g pro.
Exchanges: 1 Lean Meat, 1 Fat

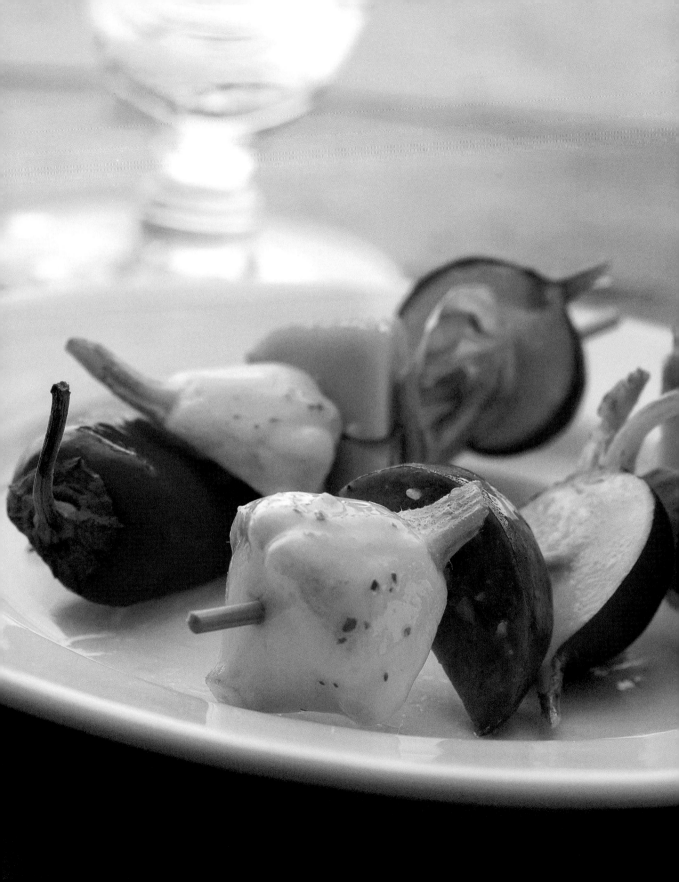

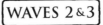

ANTIPASTO KABOBS

The variety of textures, colors, and flavors in this recipe makes it the perfect prelude to virtually any entrée. These no-cook kabobs can also be served as satisfying snacks.

Prep: 30 minutes **Marinate:** 1 to 24 hours **Makes:** 12 skewers (6 servings)

1½ to 2 cups assorted fresh vegetables (such as baby carrots, halved radishes, bell pepper squares, whole miniature bell peppers, or halved pattypan squash)

2 ounces part-skim mozzarella cheese, provolone cheese, or smoked Gouda cheese, cut into ½-inch pieces

2 ounces cooked smoked turkey sausage, cut into ¾-inch-thick slices and quartered

2 tablespoons refrigerated basil pesto

1 tablespoon white wine vinegar

12 whole fresh basil leaves

1. Place vegetables, cheese, and sausage in a self-sealing plastic bag set in a deep bowl. For marinade, in a small bowl stir together pesto and vinegar; pour over vegetable mixture. Seal bag; turn to coat vegetable mixture. Marinate in the refrigerator for 1 to 24 hours, turning bag occasionally.

2. On twelve 4-inch-long wooden skewers, alternately thread vegetables, cheese, sausage, and basil leaves.

Nutrition facts per serving: 84 cal., 6 g total fat (2 g sat. fat), 13 mg chol., 188 mg sodium, 3 g carbo., 1 g fiber, 5 g pro.
Exchanges: ½ Vegetable, ½ Lean Meat, 1 Fat

Bell Peppers

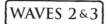 # SOY SNACKS

Each version of this fuss-free snack requires no more than 4 ingredients!
Amazingly versatile, these soybeans can be used as crunchy toppers to soups
and salads or eaten alone as a snack.

Prep: 5 minutes **Bake:** 5 minutes **Oven:** 350°F **Makes:** 2 cups

8 ounces dry roasted soybeans (2 cups)

1 recipe Spicy Thyme Seasoning Mix, Sesame-Ginger Seasoning Mix, or East India Seasoning Mix

1. Preheat oven to 350°F. Spread soybeans in an even layer on an ungreased baking sheet. Sprinkle or drizzle soybeans with Spicy Thyme Seasoning Mix, Sesame-Ginger Seasoning Mix, or East India Seasoning Mix. Toss gently.

2. Bake about 5 minutes or just until heated through, shaking pan once. Cool completely.

3. Store for up to a week in an airtight container. Eat plain, toss into soups or salads, add to hot baked potatoes, or mix with popcorn or other party mixes.

Spicy Thyme Seasoning Mix: In a small bowl combine 1½ teaspoons dried thyme, crushed; ¼ teaspoon garlic salt; and ⅛ to ¼ teaspoon cayenne pepper.

Nutrition facts per ¼-cup serving with Spicy Thyme Seasoning: 150 cal., 7 g total fat (1 g sat. fat), 0 mg chol., 33 mg sodium, 8 g carbo., 6 g fiber, 14 g pro. Exchanges: ½ Starch, 1½ Medium-Fat Meat

Sesame-Ginger Seasoning Mix: In a small bowl combine 2 teaspoons toasted sesame oil, ¾ teaspoon ground ginger, and ½ teaspoon onion salt.

Nutrition facts per ¼-cup serving with Sesame-Ginger Seasoning: 158 cal., 8 g total fat (1 g sat. fat), 0 mg chol., 103 mg sodium, 8 g carbo., 6 g fiber, 14 g pro. Exchanges: ½ Starch, 1½ Medium-Fat Meat

East India Seasoning Mix: In a small bowl combine 1½ teaspoons garam masala, ¼ teaspoon kosher salt, and ⅛ to ¼ teaspoon cayenne pepper.

Nutrition facts per ¼-cup serving with East India Seasoning: 149 cal., 7 g total fat (1 g sat. fat), 0 mg chol., 64 mg sodium, 8 g carbo., 6 g fiber, 14 g pro. Exchanges: ½ Starch, 1½ Medium-Fat Meat

SONOMA express   SPICED POPCORN

Popcorn seasoned with a blend of spices makes a delicious whole grain snack. It is also a good source of insoluble fiber.

Start to Finish: 10 minutes   **Makes:** 12 (1-cup) servings

½   teaspoon ground cumin

½   teaspoon chili powder

¼   to ½ teaspoon kosher salt

Dash cayenne pepper

Dash ground cinnamon

12 cups popped popcorn

Nonstick olive oil cooking spray

Olive Oil

Whole Grains

1. In a small bowl stir together cumin, chili powder, kosher salt, cayenne pepper, and cinnamon.

2. Spread popped popcorn in an even layer in a large shallow baking pan. Lightly coat popcorn with nonstick cooking spray. Sprinkle the cumin mixture evenly over popcorn; toss to coat.

Nutrition facts per 1-cup serving: 31 cal., 0 g total fat (0 g sat. fat), 0 mg chol., 42 mg sodium, 6 g carbo., 1 g fiber, 1 g pro.
Exchanges: ½ Starch

East Indian Spiced Popcorn: Prepare Spiced Popcorn as directed, except substitute ½ teaspoon curry powder, ½ teaspoon garam masala, ¼ teaspoon ground turmeric, and ¼ teaspoon freshly ground black pepper for the cumin, chili powder, cayenne pepper, and cinnamon.

Nutrition facts per 1-cup serving: 32 cal., 0 g total fat, 0 mg chol., 41 mg sodium, 6 g carbo., 1 g fiber, 1 g pro.
Exchanges: ½ Starch

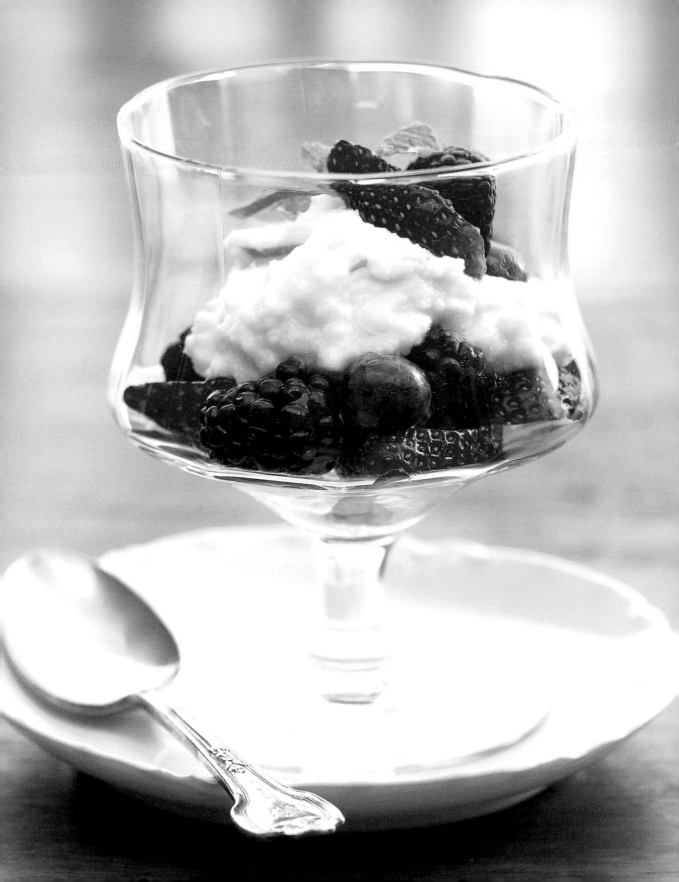

RICOTTA MOUSSE WITH BERRIES

The combination of fresh, sweet berries served over a spoonful of ricotta mousse is the perfect ending to your meal. Orange liqueur such as Grand Marnier or Bauchant adds dark citrus flavor to the mix.

Prep: 15 minutes **Chill:** 1 to 24 hours **Stand:** 15 minutes **Makes:** 4 servings

1 cup light ricotta cheese

2 tablespoons orange liqueur

½ teaspoon finely shredded orange peel

½ cup sliced fresh strawberries

½ cup fresh blueberries

½ cup fresh raspberries

½ cup fresh blackberries

1 teaspoon lemon juice

2 teaspoons honey

Fresh mint leaves (optional)

1. In a small bowl whisk together ricotta, 1 tablespoon of the orange liqueur, and the orange peel. Cover and chill for 1 to 24 hours.

2. In a medium bowl combine the berries, lemon juice, and the remaining 1 tablespoon liqueur. Cover and let stand at room temperature 15 minutes to develop flavors.

3. To serve, divide fruit mixture among four dessert dishes, spooning any juices over fruit in dishes. Top with ricotta mixture. Drizzle with honey. If desired, garnish with mint.

Nutrition facts per serving: 112 cal., 3 g total fat (2 g sat. fat), 15 mg chol., 56 mg sodium, 13 g carbo., 3 g fiber, 6 g pro.
Exchanges: ½ Fruit, ½ Other Carbo., 1 Lean Meat

Blueberries

Strawberries

POACHED PEARS IN RED WINE SAUCE

Pears poached in a brilliant red wine sauce make a most elegant and flavorful dessert.
This recipe makes enough for 6, so it's perfect fare for entertaining.

Prep: 20 minutes **Cook:** 30 minutes **Stand:** 30 minutes **Chill:** 1 to 4 hours **Makes:** 6 servings

3	medium ripe but still slightly firm pears (such as Bosc, Bartlett, or Comice)
4	cups cold water
3	tablespoons lemon juice
1½	cups port
1	cup water
⅛	teaspoon kosher salt
1	small orange
4	inches stick cinnamon
2	tablespoons honey

1. Peel pears, leaving stems intact. Cut pears in half lengthwise and scoop out the cores. Place pears in a large bowl. Add the 4 cups cold water and the lemon juice.

2. In a very large skillet combine port, the 1 cup water, and the kosher salt. Using a vegetable peeler, remove peel from the orange, being careful not to remove the white pith under the peel. If necessary, use a sharp knife to scrape off white pith from the peel. (Save orange for another use.) Add orange peel and stick cinnamon to skillet. Bring to boiling. Drain pear halves and add to skillet. Return to boiling; reduce heat. Cover and simmer about 20 minutes or just until pear halves are tender, turning pear halves once halfway through cooking. Using a slotted spoon, transfer pear halves to a shallow dish.

3. Bring poaching liquid to boiling in the same skillet. Boil gently, uncovered, for 5 to 8 minutes or until liquid is reduced to ¾ cup. Remove from heat. Stir in honey. Let liquid stand about 30 minutes or until cool. Strain liquid, discarding orange peel and stick cinnamon. Add liquid to pear halves in dish. Cover and chill for 1 to 4 hours or until completely chilled.

Nutrition facts per serving: 165 cal., 0 g total fat (0 g sat. fat), 0 mg chol., 45 mg sodium, 27 g carbo., 3 g fiber, 0 g pro.
Exchanges: 2 Fruit

HONEY-NUT SPREAD

This spreadable snack tastes great on fruit and whole grain crackers
and is as delicious as it is simple.

Start to Finish: 10 minutes **Makes:** about ⅔ cup spread

⅓ cup reduced-fat cream cheese (Neufchâtel) (about 3 ounces), softened

1 tablespoon honey

1 tablespoon chopped walnuts

⅛ teaspoon ground cinnamon or cardamom

2 tablespoons snipped dried figs, dates, or dried apricots

Low-fat milk (optional)

Graham cracker squares, apple slices, or pear slices

1. In a small bowl stir together the cream cheese, honey, walnuts, and cinnamon; stir in dried fruit.

2. If necessary, stir in 2 to 3 teaspoons milk to make desired spreading consistency. Serve with graham crackers or fruit.

Nutrition facts per 1-tablespoon spread with 2 graham cracker squares: 99 cal., 4 g total fat (2 g sat. fat), 6 mg chol., 119 mg sodium, 14 g carbo., 1 g fiber, 2 g pro.
Exchanges: 1 Starch, ½ Fat

Make-ahead directions: Prepare as directed through step 1. Cover and chill for up to 24 hours. Continue as directed.

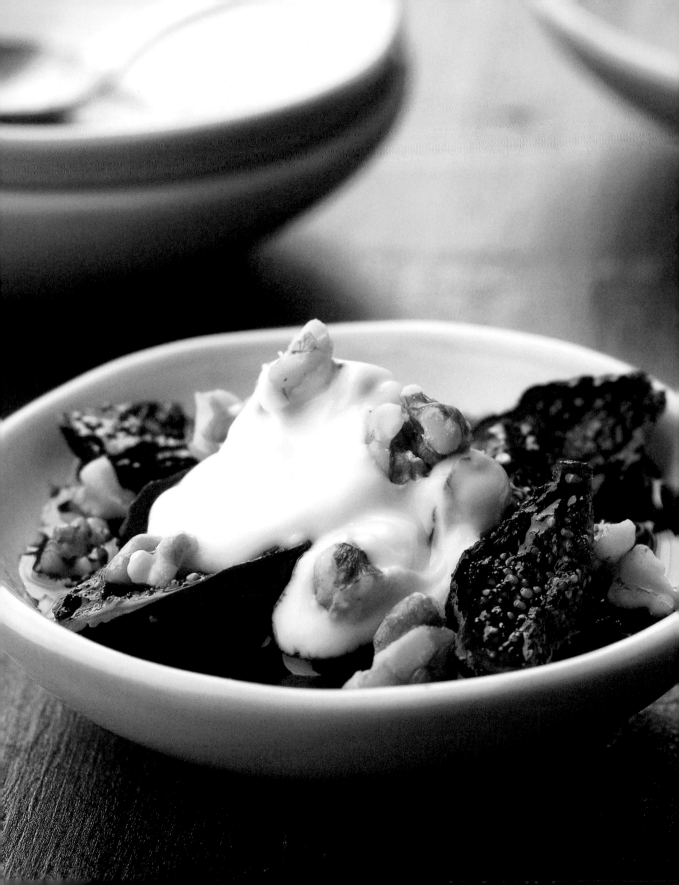

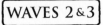
FIGS WITH PORT GLAZE

Port is a sweet fortified wine named after the Portuguese city of Oporto, where these wines are shipped from. This dessert combines port with honey and lemon juice to make a sweet glaze.

Prep: 10 minutes **Cook:** 15 minutes **Stand:** 10 minutes **Makes:** 6 servings

½ cup port

2 tablespoons honey

½ teaspoon lemon juice

Dash kosher salt

18 dried Mission figs, halved lengthwise (about 1¼ cups)

1 6-ounce carton plain low-fat yogurt

⅓ cup chopped walnuts or almonds, toasted

1. In a small saucepan combine the port, honey, lemon juice, and kosher salt. Bring to boiling; reduce heat. Boil gently, uncovered, for 15 to 20 minutes or until thickened and syrupy. Stir in figs to coat. Cover and let stand for 10 minutes.

2. Serve warm fig mixture topped with yogurt and walnuts.

Nutrition facts per serving: 256 cal., 5 g total fat (1 g sat. fat), 2 mg chol., 46 mg sodium, 48 g carbo., 6 g fiber, 4 g pro.
Exchanges: 1 Fruit, 2 Other Carbo., 1 Fat

Almonds

CITRUS FRUIT CUPS

On a hot summer day, the tropical taste of these refreshing fruit cups will hit the spot and give you a huge dose of vitamin C.

Start to Finish: 40 minutes **Makes:** 14 (½-cup) servings

4 medium pink grapefruit

3 medium oranges

3 medium tangerines

2 cups fresh strawberries

1 cup fresh blueberries

2 kiwifruits, peeled and sliced

2 limes

Fresh mint sprigs (optional)

Lime wedges (optional)

1. Peel and section grapefruit and oranges. Peel tangerines; cut tangerines into bite-size pieces. Quarter strawberries.

2. In a large bowl combine grapefruit, oranges, tangerines, and strawberries. Add blueberries and kiwifruits; toss gently.

3. Finely shred peel from the 2 limes (you should have 1 tablespoon). Squeeze lime juice (you should have ¼ cup). Gently stir lime peel and juice into fruit mixture. If desired, garnish with mint and lime wedges.

Nutrition facts per serving: 49 cal., 0 g total fat (0 g sat. fat), 0 mg chol., 1 mg sodium, 12 g carbo., 2 g fiber, 1 g pro.
Exchanges: 1 Fruit

Make-ahead directions: Prepare as directed. Cover and chill for up to 4 hours.

Blueberries   *Strawberries*

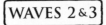
SPICED BAKED CUSTARD

Custard is a luxurious, old-fashioned way to end a meal. Easy as can be, it offers a sense of comfort with its warmth and cinnamon-like flavor from a sprinkling of allspice.

Prep: 10 minutes **Bake:** 30 minutes **Oven:** 325°F **Makes:** 4 servings

3 beaten eggs

1½ cups low-fat milk

⅓ cup heat-stable granular sugar substitute (Splenda)

1½ teaspoons vanilla

½ teaspoon ground allspice

1. Preheat oven to 325°F. In a small bowl combine eggs, milk, sugar substitute, and vanilla. Beat until combined. Place four 6-ounce custard cups in a 2-quart square baking dish. Divide egg mixture among custard cups; sprinkle with allspice. Place baking dish on oven rack. Pour boiling water into baking dish around custard cups to a depth of 1 inch.

2. Bake for 30 to 45 minutes or until a knife inserted near the center of each cup comes out clean. Remove cups from water. Cool slightly on a wire rack before serving.

Nutrition facts per serving: 99 cal., 5 g total fat (2 g sat. fat), 163 mg chol., 93 mg sodium, 7 g carbo., 0 g fiber, 8 g pro.
Exchanges: ½ Milk, ½ Medium-Fat Meat, ½ Fat

Make-ahead directions: Prepare as directed. Cool completely. Cover and chill for up to 24 hours.

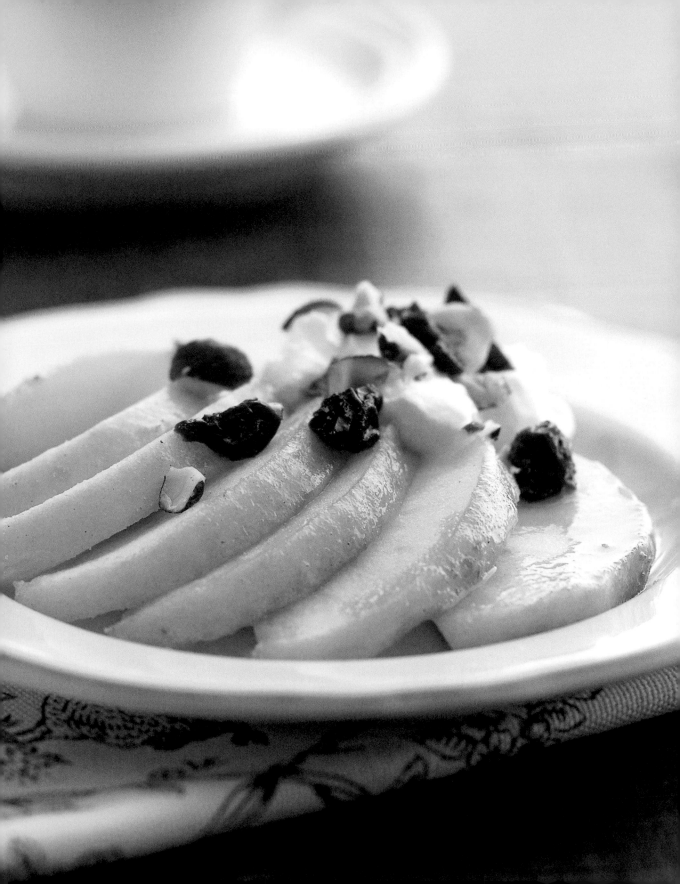

Holiday Favorites

It's time to celebrate! Here you'll find holiday foods
that are in the spirit of The Sonoma Diet and are even
more delicious and family pleasing than traditional
fare. Make Herb Roast Turkey the centerpiece of your
holiday feast. Then serve it with some Pear-Pecan
Dressing. And how about Roasted Apples with Yogurt,
Dried Cherries, and Hazelnuts for dessert?
Top it off with a glass of wine. Cheers!

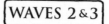

FESTIVE PITA WEDGES

These wedges make amazing appetizers for your holiday feast. With grain, vegetables, and protein all included, they are substantial enough to hold over any guest until the main meal.

Start to Finish: 25 minutes **Makes:** 32 wedges

4 large whole wheat pita bread rounds

⅓ cup bottled roasted red bell peppers, drained and chopped

3 tablespoons chopped pitted kalamata olives

1 tablespoon extra-virgin olive oil

2 cloves garlic, minced (1 teaspoon minced)

1 teaspoon chopped fresh thyme

1 teaspoon sherry vinegar

Kosher salt

Freshly ground black pepper

1 cup lightly packed arugula leaves, coarsely chopped

2 teaspoons lemon juice

4 ounces thinly sliced roast beef, cut into thin strips

2 tablespoons small shavings Parmesan cheese or Asiago cheese

1. Preheat broiler. Cut each pita round into 4 wedges. Split each wedge in half horizontally. Place wedges on one very large or two large baking sheets. Broil 4 to 5 inches from the heat for 2 to 3 minutes or until lightly toasted, turning once. Cool pita wedges on a wire rack. (If using two large baking sheets, broil one sheet at a time.)

2. In a small bowl combine roasted bell peppers, olives, olive oil, garlic, thyme, and sherry vinegar. Season to taste with kosher salt and black pepper. In another small bowl toss together the arugula and lemon juice. Season to taste with kosher salt and black pepper.

3. Divide arugula mixture among toasted pita wedges. Top with roast beef. Divide roasted pepper mixture among pita wedges, spooning over beef. Top with cheese. Serve immediately.

Nutrition facts per pita wedge: 34 cal., 1 g total fat (0 g sat. fat), 3 mg chol., 115 mg sodium, 5 g carbo., 1 g fiber, 2 g pro.
Exchanges: ½ Starch

Olive Oil   *Bell Peppers*

Whole Grains

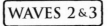
STUFFED CHERRY TOMATOES

These bite-size appetizers add a brilliant splash of red and green to your holiday table.

Start to Finish: 45 minutes **Makes:** 30 tomatoes

30 cherry tomatoes (each about 1 inch in diameter)

1 cup firmly packed fresh basil leaves

½ cup firmly packed fresh flat-leaf parsley leaves

¼ cup pine nuts, toasted

1 large clove garlic, quartered

⅛ teaspoon freshly ground black pepper

2 tablespoons extra-virgin olive oil

4 ounces goat cheese (chèvre), crumbled (1 cup)

Fresh basil leaves (optional)

Olive Oil

Tomatoes

1. Slice off the very top of each tomato. Cut a thin slice off the bottom of each tomato so it stands level. Scoop out each tomato from the top using a very small, narrow spoon. Turn upside down on paper towels to drain.

2. For pesto, in a blender or food processor combine the 1 cup basil, the parsley, pine nuts, garlic, and pepper. Cover and blend or process with several on/off turns until a paste forms, stopping machine several times and scraping the side. With the machine running slowly, gradually add olive oil through hole in lid or feed tube and blend or process until the consistency of soft butter. Transfer to a small bowl and stir in the goat cheese.

3. Spoon pesto mixture into a small self-sealing plastic bag. Snip a small hole in one corner of the bag. Seal bag. Squeeze pesto into the tomato shells. Place filled tomatoes on a serving plate. If desired, garnish with small basil leaves.

Nutrition facts per tomato: 29 cal., 2 g total fat (1 g sat. fat), 2 mg chol., 16 mg sodium, 1 g carbo., 0 g fiber, 1 g pro.
Exchanges: ½ Fat

Make-ahead directions: Prepare as directed. Cover and chill for up to 4 hours.

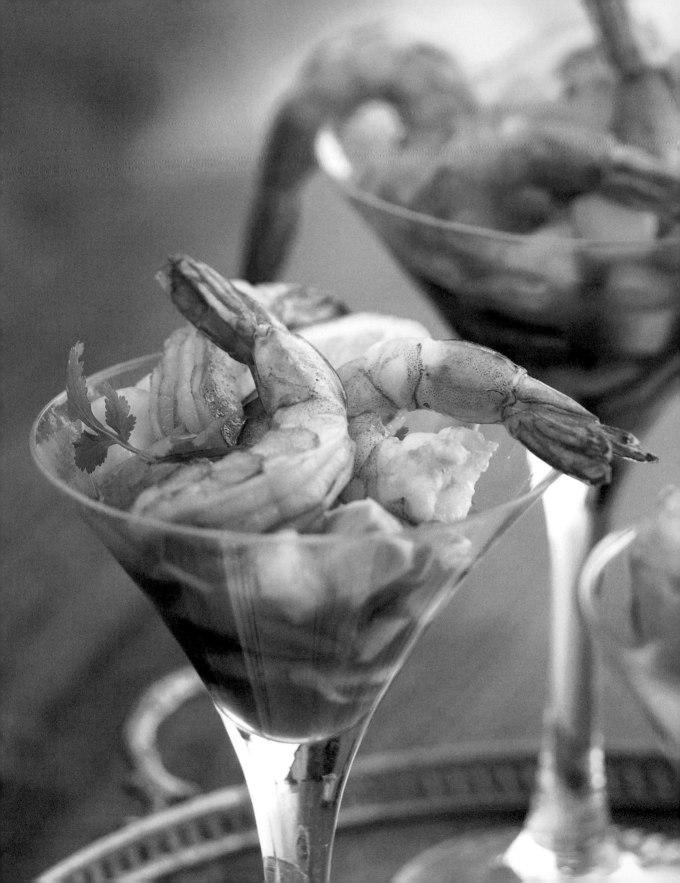

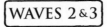

SMOKY MEXICAN SEAFOOD COCKTAIL

This festive appetizer is succulent and sweet, thanks to the starring ingredients, shrimp and crabmeat. It looks exquisite served in martini glasses but will take you only 20 minutes to prepare.

Start to Finish: 20 minutes **Makes:** 8 appetizer servings

1½ cups clam-tomato juice cocktail, chilled

½ cup finely chopped red onion

¼ cup chopped fresh cilantro

¼ cup lime juice

1 tablespoon tomato paste (optional)

1 to 2 teaspoons bottled chipotle pepper sauce or bottled hot pepper sauce

12 ounces cooked peeled and deveined shrimp with tails or two 6½-ounce cans crabmeat, drained, flaked, and cartilage removed*

1 medium avocado, halved, pitted, peeled, and chopped

1 cup chopped, seeded, peeled cucumber

8 lime wedges (optional)

Fresh cilantro (optional)

1. In a medium bowl combine clam-tomato juice cocktail, red onion, cilantro, lime juice, tomato paste (if using), and the chipotle pepper sauce.

2. Add the crabmeat (if using), avocado, and cucumber. Toss gently to coat. Divide mixture among eight martini glasses. Top with shrimp (if using). Garnish with lime wedges and cilantro if desired.

Nutrition facts per serving: 109 cal., 4 g total fat (1 g sat. fat), 65 mg chol., 233 mg sodium, 9 g carbo., 2 g fiber, 10 g pro.
Exchanges: ½ Vegetable, ½ Other Carbo., 1½ Very Lean Meat, ½ Fat

*Note: If you prefer, use a mixture of shrimp and crabmeat (12 ounces total).

Tomatoes

SHAVED FENNEL WITH ORANGES AND POMEGRANATES

This fruit and fennel salad has festive red pomegranate seeds that make this a perfect holiday side dish. And with its healthy dose of vitamin C and several phytochemicals, this is one holiday dish you can fill up on and feel good about.

Start to Finish: 40 minutes **Makes:** 8 side-dish servings

2 tablespoons red wine vinegar

2 tablespoons lemon juice

2 tablespoons extra-virgin olive oil

Kosher salt

Freshly ground black pepper

2 medium fennel bulbs

6 medium oranges, peeled and sectioned

1 cup pomegranate seeds (2 pomegranates)

¼ cup flat-leaf parsley leaves

Olive Oil

1. For vinaigrette, in a small bowl whisk together the vinegar, lemon juice, and olive oil until well mixed. Season to taste with kosher salt and pepper. Set aside.

2. Cut off and discard upper stalks from fennel bulbs. Remove any wilted outer layers and cut a thin slice from the base of each fennel bulb. Using a mandolin or sharp knife, slice fennel bulbs into very thin slices. In a large bowl combine the sliced fennel, orange sections, pomegranate seeds, and parsley leaves. Add the vinaigrette and toss gently to combine.

Tip: To avoid getting stained by the pomegranate seeds, cut the pomegranate in half and place it in a large bowl of water. Then remove the seeds. They will float to the top of the water.

Nutrition facts per serving: 122 cal., 4 g total fat (0 g sat. fat), 0 mg chol., 93 mg sodium, 23 g carbo., 4 g fiber, 2 g pro.
Exchanges: 1 Fruit, 1 Fat

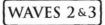
GOLDEN VEGETABLE GRATIN

A delicious fusion of sweet and savory, this richly colored vegetable dish is bursting with vitamin A. No one at your Thanksgiving feast will be able to pass up these tender, sweetly scented veggies.

Prep: 30 minutes **Bake:** 35 minutes + 10 minutes **Oven:** 375°F **Makes:** 8 side-dish servings

1 cup thinly bias-sliced carrots

3 cups peeled, quartered, and thinly sliced rutabaga (1 small)

¾ cup finely shredded Swiss cheese (3 ounces)

2½ cups peeled and thinly sliced sweet potatoes (2 medium)

2 cups peeled, quartered lengthwise, and thinly sliced butternut squash (½ of a small)

2 tablespoons water

2 tablespoons honey

½ teaspoon instant chicken bouillon granules

½ teaspoon kosher salt

¼ teaspoon freshly ground black pepper

2 tablespoons sliced almonds

1. Preheat oven to 375°F. In a 2-quart baking dish layer in order: carrots, rutabaga, ¼ cup of the cheese, the sweet potatoes, and squash. In a small bowl combine the water, honey, bouillon granules, kosher salt, and pepper; pour over vegetables.

2. Bake, covered, about 35 minutes or just until vegetables are tender. Uncover vegetables; sprinkle with the remaining ½ cup cheese and the sliced almonds. Bake, uncovered, for 10 to 15 minutes more or until almonds are lightly browned.

Nutrition facts per serving: 151 cal., 5 g total fat (2 g sat. fat), 11 mg chol., 239 mg sodium, 24 g carbo., 4 g fiber, 6 g pro.
Exchanges: ½ Vegetable, 1 Starch, ½ Medium-Fat Meat, ½ Fat

Almonds

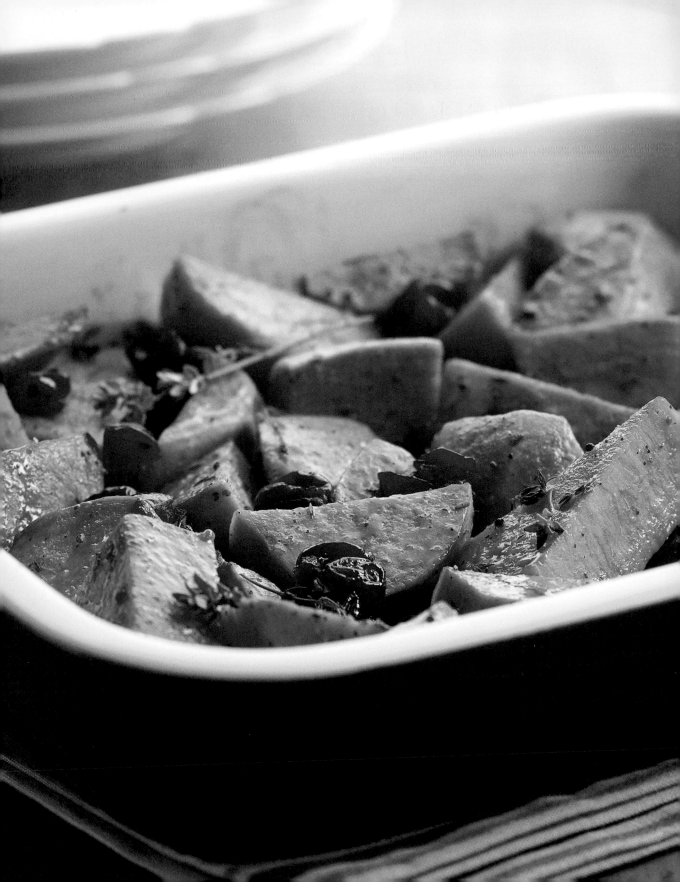

SWEET POTATO AND CRANBERRY BAKE

Sweet potatoes and cranberries always have a place at the Thanksgiving table. This stunning combination of the two essentials is deliciously seasoned and full flavored.

Prep: 25 minutes **Bake:** 1¼ hours + 10 minutes **Oven:** 350°F **Makes:** 6 servings

2 tablespoons coarse-grain mustard

1 tablespoon extra-virgin olive oil

1 tablespoon honey

1 tablespoon lemon juice

2 teaspoons chopped fresh thyme

¾ teaspoon kosher salt

¼ teaspoon freshly ground black pepper

2 pounds sweet potatoes, peeled and cut into 1½-inch chunks

½ cup fresh cranberries

Fresh thyme sprigs (optional)

1. Preheat oven to 350°F. In a large bowl combine mustard, olive oil, honey, lemon juice, thyme, kosher salt, and pepper. Add the sweet potatoes; toss to coat. Gently stir in the cranberries. Transfer sweet potato mixture to a 2-quart rectangular baking dish; spread into an even layer.

2. Bake, covered, about 1¼ hours or until sweet potatoes are tender, stirring once. Uncover and bake about 10 minutes more or just until sweet potatoes are starting to brown. If desired, garnish with thyme sprigs before serving.

Nutrition facts per serving: 171 cal., 2 g total fat (0 g sat. fat), 0 mg chol., 445 mg sodium, 35 g carbo., 5 g fiber, 2 g pro.
Exchanges: 2 Starch, ½ Fat

Olive Oil

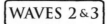
PEAR-PECAN DRESSING

The perfect side dish for any winter holiday, this delicious dressing uses warm spices and seasonings and is served hot to warm you from the inside out. The always elegant combination of fruit and nuts is sure to satisfy

Prep: 30 minutes **Bake:** 30 minutes + 15 minutes **Oven:** 350°F **Makes:** 16 side-dish servings

1   pound whole grain bread, cut into ½- to 1-inch pieces

¼   cup extra-virgin olive oil

1   cup chopped onion

1   cup chopped celery

2   medium pears, cored and chopped

1   tablespoon chopped fresh thyme

2   teaspoons chopped fresh sage

¼   teaspoon ground nutmeg

¼   teaspoon freshly ground black pepper

2   teaspoons finely shredded lemon peel

3   tablespoons lemon juice

1   cup pecans, toasted and coarsely chopped

1½   to 1¾ cups reduced-sodium chicken broth

Fresh sage (optional)

1. Preheat oven to 350°F. In a very large bowl toss bread cubes with 2 tablespoons of the olive oil. Divide bread between two shallow baking pans. Bake for 10 to 15 minutes or until golden brown and dry.

2. Meanwhile, in a large skillet heat the remaining 2 tablespoons olive oil over medium heat. Add onion and celery; cook for 5 to 8 minutes or until tender, stirring occasionally. Add the pears, thyme, sage, nutmeg, and pepper; cook for 4 minutes more, stirring occasionally. Remove from heat. Stir in lemon peel and lemon juice.

3. In a very large bowl combine toasted bread, onion mixture, and pecans. Add enough of the chicken broth to moisten. Transfer mixture to a 3-quart rectangular baking dish. Bake, covered with foil, for 30 minutes. Uncover and bake about 15 minutes more or until top is golden brown and mixture is heated through. If desired, garnish with fresh sage before serving.

Nutrition facts per serving: 160 cal., 9 g total fat (1 g sat. fat), 0 mg chol., 131 mg sodium, 18 g carbo., 5 g fiber, 4 g pro.
Exchanges: 1 Starch, 2 Fat

Olive Oil

Whole Grains

WILD RICE STUFFING

You won't need to worry about cutting bread into cubes because it's not an ingredient in this savory stuffing. This rice stuffing makes a delicious accompaniment to any meal and, because it's made with rice instead of bread, will hold together better if you decide to roast it in a bird.

Prep: 15 minutes **Cook:** 20 minutes + 25 minutes **Makes:** 8 to 10 side-dish servings

½ cup wild rice

2½ cups water

½ cup long grain brown rice

1 tablespoon instant chicken bouillon granules

¼ teaspoon ground sage or nutmeg

3 cups sliced fresh mushrooms

1 cup chopped celery

6 green onions, sliced

½ cup slivered almonds, toasted (optional)

1. Rinse wild rice in a strainer under cold water about 1 minute. In a large saucepan combine wild rice, the water, uncooked brown rice, bouillon granules, and sage or nutmeg. Bring to boiling; reduce heat. Cover and simmer for 20 minutes.

2. Stir in mushrooms, celery, and green onions. Cover and cook over medium-low heat about 25 minutes or just until wild rice and vegetables are tender, stirring frequently. If desired, garnish with toasted almonds. Serve immediately.

Nutrition facts per serving: 96 cal., 1 g total fat (0 g sat. fat), 0 mg chol., 340 mg sodium, 19 g carbo., 2 g fiber, 4 g pro.
Exchanges: ½ Vegetable, 1 Starch

Almonds

Whole Grains

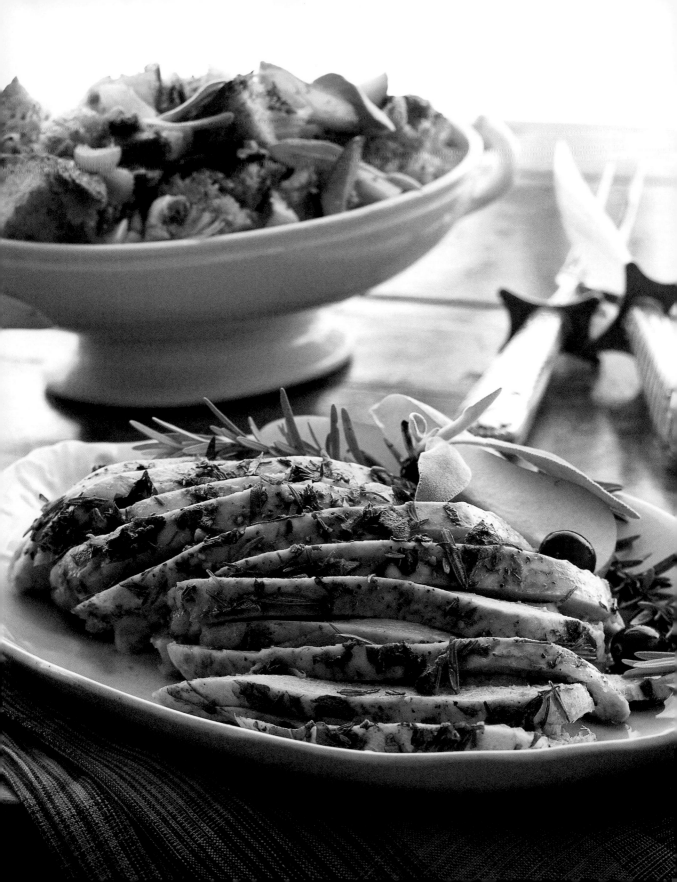

HERB ROAST TURKEY

Perfectly seasoned with a variety of spices and herbs and a dash of white wine, this roasted turkey breast makes an elegant entrée.

Prep: 20 minutes **Roast:** 15 minutes + 25 minutes **Oven:** 400°F/350°F **Makes:** 8 servings

1 2-pound boneless turkey breast, skinned

½ teaspoon kosher salt

½ teaspoon freshly ground black pepper

2 teaspoons finely shredded lemon peel

3 tablespoons lemon juice

2 tablespoons extra-virgin olive oil

1 tablespoon chopped fresh flat-leaf parsley

1 tablespoon chopped fresh rosemary

1 tablespoon chopped fresh sage

1 tablespoon chopped fresh thyme

6 cloves garlic, minced (1 tablespoon minced)

1 cup chicken broth

¼ cup dry white wine

1 tablespoon chopped fresh flat-leaf parsley

1. Preheat oven to 400°F. Season turkey breast with kosher salt and pepper. Place turkey in a shallow roasting pan. In a small bowl combine lemon peel, lemon juice, olive oil, 1 tablespoon parsley, the rosemary, sage, thyme, and garlic. Rub herb mixture over turkey breast.

2. Roast turkey for 15 minutes. Pour broth and wine over turkey. Reduce oven temperature to 350°F. Roast turkey about 25 minutes more or until turkey is tender and no longer pink (170°F), spooning juices in pan over turkey every 10 minutes.

3. To serve, slice turkey. Spoon some of the cooking juices from the roasting pan over individual servings. Sprinkle with 1 tablespoon parsley.

Nutrition facts per serving: 170 cal., 4 g total fat (1 g sat. fat), 71 mg chol., 284 mg sodium, 2 g carbo., 0 g fiber, 28 g pro.
Exchanges: 4 Very Lean Meat, 1 Fat

Wine Pairing: sparkling Pinot Noir

Olive Oil

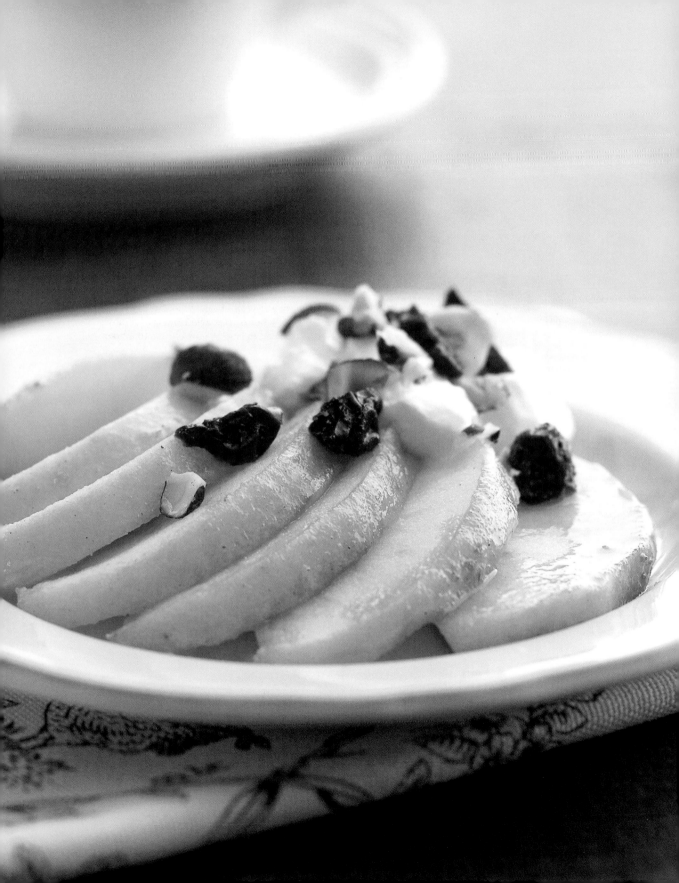

ROASTED APPLES WITH YOGURT, DRIED CHERRIES, AND HAZELNUTS

A holiday meal without dessert just wouldn't be complete, so use this dish to satisfy everyone's sweet tooth. Don't forget to plan ahead, the yogurt cheese needs at least 24 hours of refrigeration.

Prep: 15 minutes **Chill:** 24 hours **Bake:** 30 minutes **Oven:** 350°F **Makes:** 4 servings

¾ cup plain low-fat yogurt*

Nonstick olive oil cooking spray

1 teaspoon lemon juice

1 teaspoon honey

¼ teaspoon ground cinnamon

⅛ teaspoon kosher salt

2 Granny Smith apples, peeled, cored, and halved

2 tablespoons chopped hazelnuts, toasted**

1 tablespoon snipped dried cherries

1. For yogurt cheese, line a sieve or small colander with three layers of 100%-cotton cheesecloth or a clean paper coffee filter. Suspend the lined sieve or colander over a bowl. (Or use a yogurt strainer.) Spoon yogurt into sieve or colander. Cover with plastic wrap. Refrigerate for at least 24 hours. Remove from refrigerator; discard liquid. Transfer yogurt cheese to a bowl; set aside.

2. Preheat oven to 350°F. Lightly coat a small baking sheet with nonstick cooking spray; set aside. In a small bowl combine lemon juice, honey, cinnamon, and kosher salt. Brush lemon juice mixture onto apple halves. Place apple halves, cut sides down, on prepared baking sheet.

3. Bake about 30 minutes or until apple halves are lightly browned and tender. Transfer apple halves to a cutting board. Thinly slice each apple half. Divide apple slices among four dessert plates, fanning the slices on each plate. Serve with yogurt cheese; sprinkle with hazelnuts and dried cherries.

Nutrition facts per serving: 100 cal., 3 g total fat (1 g sat. fat), 3 mg chol., 93 mg sodium, 16 g carbo., 2 g fiber, 3 g pro.
Exchanges: ½ Fruit, ½ Other Carbo., ½ Fat

*Note: Use a brand of yogurt that contains no gums, gelatin, or fillers. These ingredients may prevent the whey from separating from the curd to make yogurt cheese.

**Note: To toast the hazelnuts, preheat oven to 350°F. Place the nuts in a shallow baking pan. Bake about 10 minutes or until toasted. Place the warm nuts on a clean kitchen towel. Rub the nuts with the towel to remove the loose skins.

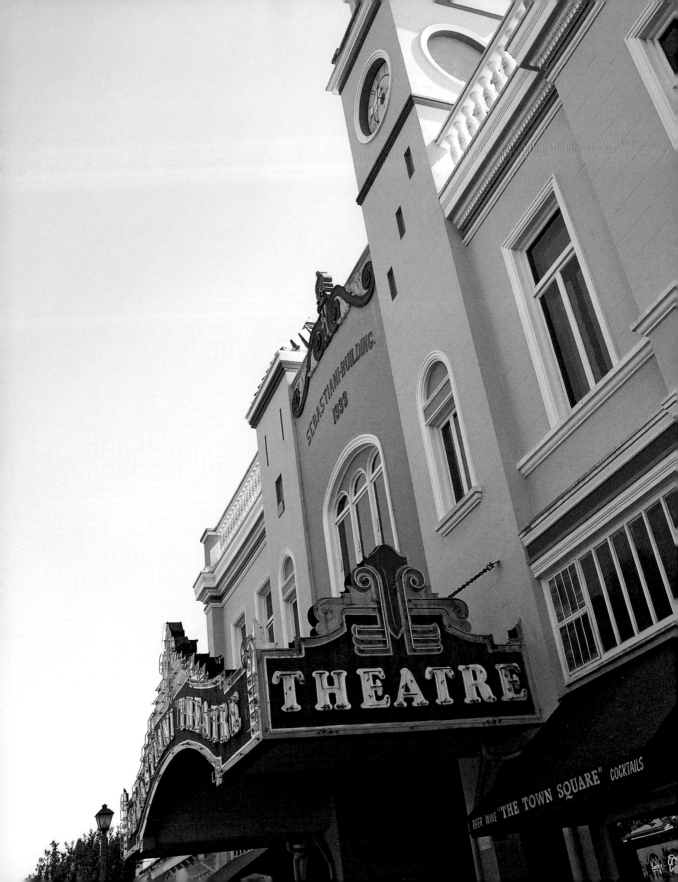

Taste of Sonoma

Enjoy the rich flavors of Sonoma County in your own kitchen with these inspired recipes. Provided by chefs at various local Sonoma inns, restaurants, and wineries, these dishes give you the wine country flavors that make this region such a sought-after destination.

FIG SALAD WITH FIG AND PORT VINAIGRETTE

This fig salad, which has become our most popular signature dish, encompasses wine country simply by combining ingredients that are significant alone and when combined create a uniquely delicious flavor. These are the fruits of the earth and of the wine country territory.

Start to Finish: 50 minutes **Makes:** 8 side-dish servings

2 ounces pancetta, chopped

1 tablespoon extra-virgin olive oil

12 fresh figs, halved, or 6 plums (2 pounds), pitted and quartered

8 cups arugula

½ cup pecan halves, toasted

4 ounces semisoft goat cheese (chèvre), crumbled

¾ cup Fig and Port Vinaigrette

Freshly ground black pepper

1. In a 10-inch skillet cook and stir the pancetta over medium heat until crisp. Remove with a slotted spoon and set aside, reserving drippings in skillet. Add olive oil to skillet. Add the figs or plums to skillet. Cook the figs about 2 minutes or until slightly softened and browned, turning once. (Or cook the plums about 5 minutes or until slightly softened and browned, turning once.)

2. In a very large bowl toss together the cooked pancetta, arugula, pecans, goat cheese, and Fig and Port Vinaigrette. Divide the greens mixture among eight salad plates; surround greens with figs or plums. Sprinkle individual servings lightly with pepper.

Nutrition facts per serving: 308 cal., 22 g total fat (4 g sat. fat), 12 mg chol., 219 mg sodium, 21 g carbo., 4 g fiber, 5 g pro.
Exchanges: 1 Vegetable, ½ Fruit, ½ Other Carbo., ½ Medium-Fat Meat, 4 Fat

Fig and Port Vinaigrette: In a small saucepan combine 3 dried Mission figs and 1 cup port; let stand at room temperature for 30 minutes. Using a slotted spoon, transfer figs to a blender; set aside. Heat port to boiling over medium-high heat; reduce heat. Boil gently, uncovered, for 8 to 10 minutes or until reduced to ½ cup. Cool slightly; add to blender along with ¼ cup red wine vinegar. Cover and blend until figs are very finely chopped. With the blender running, add ¾ cup canola oil in a slow, steady stream; blend until well mixed and thickened. Stop blender. Add 2 teaspoons finely chopped shallots, ¼ teaspoon kosher salt, and ⅛ teaspoon freshly ground black pepper; cover and blend for 5 seconds more. Serve immediately or cover and chill for up to 5 days. Makes about 1½ cups.

Source: The Girl & the Fig Cookbook

HEARTS OF PALM, AVOCADO, AND RED ONION SALAD WITH CORIANDER VINAIGRETTE

This recipe and the others from The Culinary Institute of America were originally created by Catherine Brandel, who was an incredible chef with an amazing passion for food and agriculture. She taught many chefs the importance of using seasonal ingredients from local farms. She always instilled the importance of flavor, taste, and quality, as you'll see in this simple salad recipe.

Start to Finish: 25 minutes **Makes:** 8 side-dish servings

2 tablespoons chopped fresh cilantro

2 tablespoons lime juice

1 clove garlic, minced (½ teaspoon minced)

¼ cup extra-virgin olive oil

1 14-ounce can or jar hearts of palm, drained and cut into 1-inch-thick slices

1 avocado, halved, seeded, peeled, and cut into bite-size pieces

1 cup cherry tomatoes, halved, or 1 cup coarsely chopped roma tomatoes

¼ cup thinly sliced red onion

1 head butterhead (Boston or Bibb) lettuce, trimmed and torn (6 cups)

Freshly cracked black pepper

1. For vinaigrette, in a small bowl combine cilantro, lime juice, and garlic. Add olive oil in a thin, steady stream, whisking constantly until mixture is well mixed and slightly thickened. Set aside.

2. In a large bowl combine hearts of palm, avocado, tomatoes, and red onion. Add vinaigrette; toss gently to coat.

3. To serve, divide lettuce among eight salad plates. Mound tomato mixture on top of lettuce. Sprinkle with cracked black pepper.

Nutrition facts per serving: 117 cal., 10 g total fat (1 g sat. fat), 0 mg chol., 203 mg sodium, 6 g carbo., 3 g fiber, 2 g pro.
Exchanges: 1 Vegetable, 2 Fat

Source: Toni Sakaguchi, Chef Instructor at The Culinary Institute of America In honor of Chef Catherine Brandel, Chef Instructor at The Culinary Institute of America

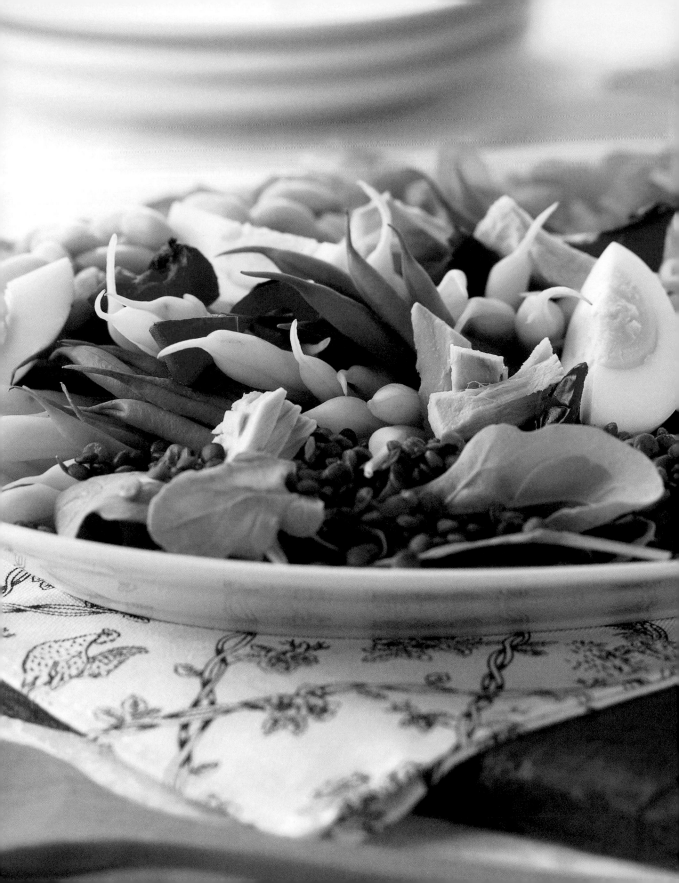

THREE-BEAN, LENTIL, AND ARUGULA SALAD WITH GRILLED RED PEPPERS AND HERB VINAIGRETTE

With its bright colors and fresh ingredients, this main dish salad is great to serve when entertaining. It tastes best when served at room temperature rather than chilled.

Prep: 45 minutes **Cook:** 30 minutes **Grill:** 10 minutes **Makes:** 8 servings

⅔ cup dry green or brown lentils

2 cups water

2 red bell peppers

1 pound fresh haricots verts (green beans), trimmed if desired

1 pound fresh haricots beurres (yellow wax beans), trimmed if desired

1 cup fresh flat-leaf parsley leaves

¾ cup lightly packed fresh basil leaves

¼ cup lightly packed fresh mint leaves

¼ cup white balsamic vinegar

2 shallots, coarsely chopped

¾ cup extra-virgin olive oil

Kosher salt

Freshly ground black pepper

8 cups arugula

1 19-ounce can cannellini beans (white kidney beans), rinsed and drained

1 9-ounce can solid white tuna (water pack), drained and broken into chunks

4 hard-cooked eggs, peeled and cut into wedges

2 to 3 tablespoons capers, drained (optional)

1. Rinse and pick over lentils. In a large saucepan bring the water to boiling; add lentils. Return to boiling; reduce heat. Cover and simmer about 30 minutes or until lentils are tender; drain and set aside.

2. Cut bell peppers lengthwise into quarters, removing stems and seeds. For a charcoal grill,° place pepper quarters on the rack of an uncovered grill directly over medium coals. Grill for 10 to 12 minutes or just until beginning to char, turning once halfway through grilling. (For a gas grill, preheat grill. Reduce heat to medium. Place pepper quarters on grill rack over heat. Cover and grill as above.) Transfer pepper quarters to a cutting board. Coarsely chop peppers; set aside.

3. In a covered large Dutch oven cook fresh beans in a small amount of lightly salted boiling water for 4 to 5 minutes or just until tender. (If using frozen beans, cook according to package directions.) Drain; immediately plunge into ice water to cool quickly. When cool, drain well.

4. For vinaigrette, in a blender combine parsley, basil, mint, vinegar, and shallots. Cover and blend until herbs and shallots are finely chopped. With blender or food processor running, slowly add the olive oil in a thin, steady stream; blend or process until well mixed. Season to taste with kosher salt and black pepper. Set aside.

5. To serve, place the arugula leaves down the two long sides of a large platter. Top one side of the arugula with the cannellini beans. Top the other side of the arugula with the lentils. Down the center alternately crisscross small bundles of the green and yellow beans (or arrange combined beans down the center). Top the green and yellow beans with the chopped bell pepper. Top salad with the tuna and egg wedges. Drizzle with some of the herb vinaigrette; pass remaining vinaigrette. If desired sprinkle with the capers.

Nutrition facts per serving: 409 cal., 25 g total fat (4 g sat. fat), 119 mg chol., 336 mg sodium, 32 g carbo., 13 g fiber, 22 g pro.
Exchanges: 1 Starch, 2½ Vegetable, 2 Lean Meat, 3½ Fat

*Note: For quicker preparation, omit grilling and just coarsely chop the bell peppers.

For Wave 1, serve as is. For Waves 2 and 3, serve with fresh pear slices.

Source: Ramekins Culinary School

SPRING TABBOULEH WITH COUSCOUS

This simple side dish is light, fresh, and full of color, making it a favorite at COPIA: The American Center for Wine, Food and the Arts. COPIA is a nonprofit discovery center whose mission is to explore and celebrate the cultural significance of wine, food gardens, and the arts.

Start to Finish: 30 minutes **Makes:** 8 to 10 side-dish servings

1 cup whole wheat couscous*

1 tablespoon extra-virgin olive oil

8 ounces fresh asparagus, trimmed and cut into 1-inch-long pieces (1 cup)

½ cup chopped fennel bulb

½ cup chopped carrot

¼ cup sliced green onions

½ cup canned fava beans, rinsed and drained

3 tablespoons lemon juice

2 tablespoons extra-virgin olive oil

½ cup chopped fresh mint

½ cup chopped fresh flat-leaf parsley

Kosher salt

Freshly ground black pepper

1. In a medium saucepan bring 2 cups lightly salted water to boiling. Stir in couscous. Remove from heat. Cover and set aside to cool.

2. Meanwhile, in a large skillet heat the 1 tablespoon olive oil over medium heat. Add asparagus, fennel, carrot, and green onions; cook for 5 to 7 minutes or until vegetables are crisp-tender. Stir in fava beans. Set aside.

3. In a small bowl whisk together lemon juice and the 2 tablespoons olive oil. Place couscous in a large bowl. Add vegetable mixture, lemon juice mixture, mint, and parsley. Stir gently to combine. Season to taste with kosher salt and pepper.

Nutrition facts per serving: 177 cal., 6 g total fat (1 g sat. fat), 0 mg chol., 145 mg sodium, 28 g carbo., 5 g fiber, 6 g pro.
Exchanges: 1½ Starch, 1 Fat

*Note: Israeli couscous can be substituted for the whole wheat couscous. Cook according to package directions, draining if necessary. Israeli couscous may be hard to find in a typical supermarket, but it's at many smaller specialty stores and, any place specializing in Middle Eastern ingredients.

Source: COPIA: The American Center for Wine, Food and the Arts, Napa, California

RATATOUILLE NIÇOISE

This versatile side dish recipe from The Fairmont Sonoma Mission Inn is full of fresh vegetables and herbs. Serve it with most any meat, poultry, or fish or enjoy it as a light meatless meal.

Start to Finish: 40 minutes **Makes:** 8 side-dish servings

2 tablespoons extra-virgin olive oil

1 medium eggplant, peeled and chopped

1 medium onion, chopped

6 cloves garlic, minced (1 tablespoon minced)

3 medium green, red, and/or yellow bell peppers, seeded and chopped

1 medium yellow summer squash, chopped

1 medium zucchini, chopped

3 medium roma tomatoes, chopped

1 teaspoon chopped fresh thyme

⅛ to ¼ teaspoon cayenne pepper

   Kosher salt

   Freshly ground black pepper

½ cup chopped fresh basil

   Fresh basil leaves (optional)

1. In a 4-quart Dutch oven heat olive oil over medium-high heat. Add eggplant; cook about 3 minutes or until tender and golden brown. Add onion and garlic; cook and stir for 2 minutes. Add bell peppers; cook and stir for 2 minutes. Add summer squash and zucchini; cook and stir for 2 minutes. Add tomatoes, thyme, and cayenne pepper. Season to taste with kosher salt and black pepper. Cook and stir for 2 to 5 minutes more or until vegetables are tender. Stir in basil. Serve hot, cooled to room temperature, or chilled. If desired, garnish with fresh basil.

Nutrition facts per serving: 74 cal., 4 g total fat (1 g sat. fat), 0 mg chol., 68 mg sodium, 10 g carbo., 4 g fiber, 2 g pro.
Exchanges: 2 Vegetable, ½ Fat

Source: Chef Bruno Tison,
The Fairmont Sonoma Mission Inn

Wine Pairing: Hanzell Pinot Noir, Deerfield Ranch Chardonnay

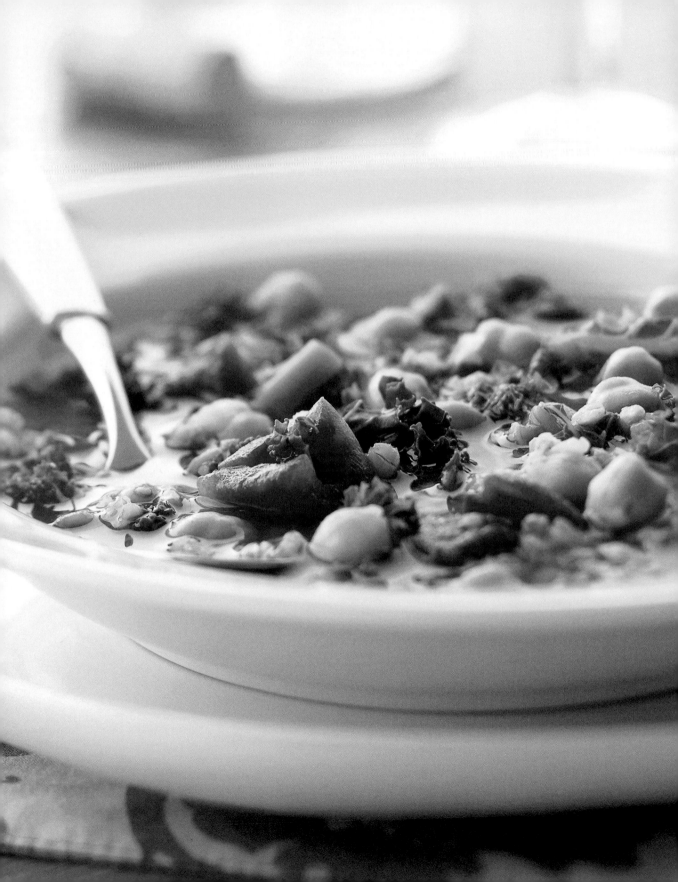

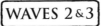

RUSTIC GARBANZO BEAN, SPELT, AND KALE SOUP

This flavor-rich soup recipe comes from Ramekins Culinary School, located in the heart of Sonoma Valley. It's hearty enough for a full meal and is great with a slice of whole grain bread.

Prep: 15 minutes **Cook:** 1 hour **Makes:** 6 to 8 servings

8 cups vegetable stock or vegetable broth

¾ cup whole spelt (farro) or regular pearl barley, rinsed and drained

1 15- to 16-ounce can garbanzo beans (chickpeas), rinsed and drained

1 14½-ounce can diced tomatoes, undrained

1 cup dry white wine

8 cloves garlic, thinly sliced

3 sprigs fresh thyme

1 tablespoon fennel seeds, crushed

6 cups coarsely chopped fresh kale leaves

½ to 1 teaspoon crushed red pepper

3 tablespoons lemon juice

Freshly ground black pepper (optional)

Chopped fresh flat-leaf parsley (optional)

1. In a 4- to 6-quart Dutch oven bring the vegetable stock to boiling. Add spelt or barley. Return to boiling; reduce heat. Cover and simmer for 25 minutes.

2. Add garbanzo beans, undrained tomatoes, wine, garlic, thyme, and fennel seeds to Dutch oven. Bring to boiling; reduce heat. Cover and simmer for 20 minutes. Add kale and crushed red pepper. Cook, uncovered, about 15 minutes or until kale and spelt are tender, stirring occasionally.

3. Stir in lemon juice. If desired, season to taste with black pepper. Remove thyme sprigs before serving. If desired, sprinkle individual servings with parsley.

Nutrition facts per serving: 278 cal., 2 g total fat (0 g sat. fat), 0 mg chol., 1,635 mg sodium, 50 g carbo., 8 g fiber, 10 g pro.
Exchanges: 1½ Vegetable, 2½ Starch, ½ Fat

Source: Chef Mary Karlin, Ramekins Culinary School

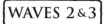
ORGANIC MUSHROOM RISOTTO

The Fairmont Sonoma Mission Inn uses a local Sebastopol mushroom variety in the recipe, but you can substitute any of the wild mushrooms suggested below. Although most risottos use rice, this version is made with barley.

Start to Finish: 40 minutes **Makes:** 8 side-dish servings

12 ounces Sebastopol organic mushrooms or other wild mushrooms (such as cinnamon cap, nameko, clam shell, baby blue oyster, shiitake, and/or cremini)

4½ to 5 cups chicken stock or chicken broth

½ cup chopped onion

6 cloves garlic, minced (1 tablespoon minced)

2 tablespoons extra-virgin olive oil

1 11-ounce box quick-cooking barley (2 cups)

1 cup dry white wine

1 ounce Parmigiano-Reggiano cheese, grated

Ground white pepper or freshly ground black pepper

Fresh chervil (optional)

1. Remove stems from mushrooms and set aside. Slice mushroom caps. In a medium saucepan combine the mushroom stems and chicken stock. Bring to boiling; reduce heat. Cover and simmer for 10 minutes. Strain stock, discarding mushroom stems. Return stock to saucepan and keep warm over low heat.

2. In a 4-quart Dutch oven cook onion and garlic in hot olive oil until tender, stirring occasionally. Add the uncooked barley; cook and stir for 2 minutes. Add wine; cook and stir until most of the liquid is absorbed. Add 1 cup of the hot stock. Cook, uncovered, until most of the stock is absorbed, stirring frequently. Continue adding stock, 1 cup at a time, cooking after each addition until stock is nearly absorbed, stirring frequently. When barley is nearly tender, quit adding stock and stop cooking. (Total cooking time should be 12 to 15 minutes after the wine is added.) Add mushroom caps. Cook and stir for 3 to 5 minutes or until mushrooms are tender.

3. Stir in the cheese. Season to taste with pepper. If desired, garnish with chervil.

Nutrition facts per serving: 246 cal., 5 g total fat (1 g sat. fat), 3 mg chol., 328 mg sodium, 39 g carbo., 5 g fiber, 8 g pro.
Exchanges: ½ Vegetable, 2½ Starch, 1 Fat

Source: Chef Richard
The Fairmont Sonoma Mission Inn

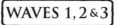
HERB-RUBBED SALMON WITH SHAVED VEGETABLE SALAD

Another favorite at the Culinary Institute of America, this recipe actually makes two dishes—a simple-to-make, yet delicious main dish salmon served with a refreshing side-dish salad.

Prep: 25 minutes **Chill:** 1 to 2 hours **Cook:** 8 minutes **Makes:** 4 servings

4 fresh or frozen skinless salmon fillets (1 to 1½ pounds total)

Kosher salt

Freshly ground black pepper

1 tablespoon chopped fresh tarragon

1 tablespoon chopped fresh chives

1 tablespoon chopped fresh flat-leaf parsley

1 tablespoon chopped fresh chervil

1 tablespoon lemon juice

1 clove garlic, minced (½ teaspoon minced)

1 recipe Shaved Vegetable Salad

1 tablespoon extra-virgin olive oil

1. Thaw salmon, if frozen. Season salmon with kosher salt and pepper. Place salmon in a 3-quart rectangular baking dish; set aside. In a small bowl combine tarragon, chives, parsley, chervil, lemon juice, and garlic. Sprinkle herb mixture over both sides of each salmon fillet; rub in with your fingers. Cover and chill for 1 to 2 hours.

2. Just before serving, prepare Shaved Vegetable Salad; set aside. In a very large skillet heat olive oil over medium-high heat. Add salmon fillets. Cook for 8 to 12 minutes or until salmon flakes easily when tested with a fork, carefully turning fillets once halfway through cooking. Turn heat down if salmon browns too much.

3. Toss Shaved Vegetable Salad to coat with vinaigrette. Divide salad among four dinner plates. Top with salmon.

Shaved Vegetable Salad: For vinaigrette, in a small bowl combine 3 tablespoons lemon juice and 1 tablespoon finely chopped shallot. Let stand for 10 minutes. Whisk in ¼ cup extra-virgin olive oil. Season to taste with kosher salt and freshly ground black pepper. Meanwhile, in a covered medium saucepan cook 1 cup 1- to 2-inch-long pieces fresh green beans in a small amount of lightly salted boiling water for 4 to 6 minutes or until crisp-tender. Drain; immediately plunge into ice water to cool quickly. Drain well. In a large bowl combine green beans, 1 cup very thinly sliced fennel bulb,° 1 cup very thinly sliced celery,° 1 cup very thinly sliced English cucumber,° 1 cup very thinly sliced zucchini,° ½ cup very thinly sliced radishes,° and ¼ cup very thinly sliced red onion.° Add the vinaigrette; toss gently to combine. Season to taste with kosher salt and freshly ground black pepper.

Nutrition facts per serving: 399 cal., 29 g total fat (5 g sat. fat), 66 mg chol., 416 mg sodium, 10 g carbo., 3 g fiber, 25 g pro.
Exchanges: 1½ Vegetable, 3 Lean Meat, 4 Fat

*Note: Use a mandoline to very thinly slice the larger vegetables and a food processor with a thin slicing blade to very thinly slice the smaller vegetables. Or use a knife to very thinly slice all of the vegetables.

For Wave 1, serve with cooked barley. For Waves 2 and 3, serve with cooked barley and fresh berries.

Source: Toni Sakaguchi, Chef Instructor at The Culinary Institute of America
In honor of Chef Catherine Brandel, Chef Instructor at The Culinary Institute of America

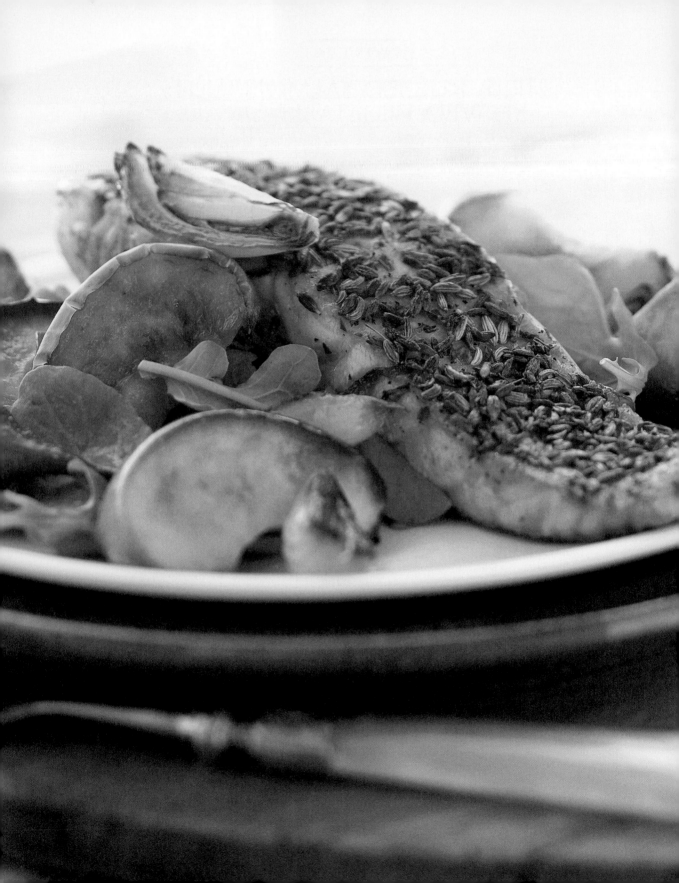

LAVENDER AND FENNEL-CRUSTED BODEGA BAY SALMON WITH SLOW-ROASTED BEETS AND HEIRLOOM APPLES

The reason Sonoma is the best playground for chefs is that its local ingredients are so pristine—they come to a chef just hours out of the earth or ocean. This recipe combines salmon fresh from Bodega Bay with lavender from the garden and heirloom apples picked just down the road.

Prep: 25 minutes **Roast:** 45 minutes **Cook:** 7 minutes + 8 minutes **Oven:** 400°F **Makes:** 6 servings

6	6-ounce fresh or frozen skinless salmon fillets, about 1 inch thick
1 ½	pounds baby beets or medium beets
4	tablespoons extra-virgin olive oil
	Kosher salt
	Freshly ground black pepper
3	medium heirloom apples or cooking apples, cored and each cut into 6 wedges
3	medium shallots, peeled and each cut into 8 wedges
2	tablespoons chopped fresh flat-leaf parsley
1	tablespoon dried lavender, crushed
2	teaspoons fennel seeds
1	teaspoon chopped fresh thyme
½	teaspoon kosher salt
½	teaspoon freshly ground black pepper
1	5-ounce package baby arugula or arugula, torn (about 6 cups)
3	tablespoons lemon juice

1. Thaw salmon, if frozen. Rinse salmon; pat dry with paper towels.

2. Preheat oven to 400°F. Trim greens from beets, if present. If using medium beets, peel beets and cut into 1-inch wedges. Place baby beets or beet wedges in a 2-quart baking dish. Drizzle with 1 tablespoon of the olive oil; season with kosher salt and pepper. Cover with foil. Roast for 45 to 50 minutes or until tender. If using baby beets, cool slightly; peel beets. Season beets with kosher salt and pepper.

3. Meanwhile, in a very large skillet heat 1 tablespoon of the remaining olive oil over medium-high heat. Add apples and shallots; cook about 7 minutes or until golden brown. Remove from skillet; cover and keep warm.

4. In a small bowl combine parsley, lavender, fennel seeds, thyme, the ½ teaspoon kosher salt, and the ½ teaspoon pepper. Sprinkle mixture evenly over one side of each salmon fillet; rub in with your fingers.

5. In the same skillet heat 1 tablespoon of the remaining olive oil over medium-high heat. Add salmon; cook for 8 to 12 minutes or until golden brown and fish just flakes easily when tested with a fork, turning once halfway through cooking.

6. In a large bowl toss the arugula with lemon juice and the remaining 1 tablespoon olive oil. Season with additional kosher salt and pepper. Divide arugula among six dinner plates. Top with beets, apple and shallot mixture, and salmon.

Nutrition facts per serving: 492 cal., 28 g total fat (5 g sat. fat), 99 mg chol., 520 mg sodium, 24 g carbo., 6 g fiber, 37 g pro.
Exchanges: 2½ Vegetable, ½ Fruit, 4½ Very Lean Meat, 3 Fat

For Wave 1, this is not appropriate. For Waves 2 and 3, serve with whole wheat bread.

Source: Chef Duskie, Cafe ZaZu

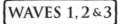
GRILLED AHI TUNA WITH RUSTIC MEDITERRANEAN SAUCE

In this recipe from St. Francis Winery in Sonoma, grilled tuna is topped with an interesting sauce that combines prepared marinara sauce with traditional Mediterrean ingredients.

Prep: 20 minutes **Cook:** 15 minutes **Grill:** 8 minutes **Makes:** 6 servings

6 fresh or frozen tuna steaks, cut 1 inch thick (about 1½ pounds total)

2 tablespoons extra-virgin olive oil

¼ teaspoon kosher salt

⅛ teaspoon freshly ground black pepper

½ cup chopped onion

6 cloves garlic, minced (1 tablespoon minced)

1 cup prepared marinara sauce

½ cup oil-packed dried tomatoes, drained and chopped

¼ cup bottled roasted red bell peppers, chopped

¼ cup golden raisins

¼ cup pitted kalamata olives, chopped

1 tablespoon chopped fresh flat-leaf parsley

1. Thaw fish, if frozen. Rinse fish; pat dry with paper towels. Brush tuna steaks with 1 tablespoon of the olive oil. Season with kosher salt and pepper; set aside.

2. For sauce, in a small saucepan heat the remaining 1 tablespoon olive oil over medium heat. Add onion and garlic; cook until tender. Stir in marinara sauce, dried tomatoes, roasted red bell peppers, raisins, and olives. Bring to boiling; reduce heat. Simmer, uncovered, for 15 minutes.

3. Meanwhile, for a charcoal grill, place fish on the greased rack of an uncovered grill directly over medium coals. Grill for 8 to 12 minutes or just until fish starts to flake when tested with a fork and center is still slightly pink, gently turning once halfway through grilling. (For a gas grill, preheat grill. Reduce heat to medium. Place fish on greased grill rack over heat. Cover and grill as above.)

4. To serve, spoon the sauce over the fish. Sprinkle with parsley.

Nutrition facts per serving: 255 cal., 9 g total fat (1 g sat. fat), 51 mg chol., 413 mg sodium, 15 g carbo., 2 g fiber, 28 g pro.
Exchanges: ½ Vegetable, 1 Other Carbo., 4 Very Lean Meat, 1½ Fat

Tip: This sauce also goes well with other white fish, chicken, or pork.

For Wave 1, serve with cooked multigrain pasta and cooked broccoli or cauliflower. For Waves 2 and 3, serve with cooked multigrain pasta, cooked broccoli or cauliflower, and fresh orange slices.

Source: Chef Todd Muir, St. Francis Winery, Sonoma, California

Wine Pairing: St. Francis Merlot

CHILE-CRUSTED LAMB WITH CUCUMBER YOGURT

The chefs at Windsor Vineyards say that the spice on the lamb lends itself beautifully to the spice in a Zinfandel wine. The Cucumber Yogurt cools the higher alcohol levels common in Zinfandel.

Prep: 25 minutes **Broil:** 10 minutes **Makes:** 4 servings

8 5-ounce lamb loin or rib chops, cut 1 inch thick

4 large fresh red jalapeño chile peppers, seeded and coarsely chopped*

½ cup fresh cilantro leaves

2 green onions, cut up

2 tablespoons lemon juice

1 tablespoon extra-virgin olive oil

⅛ teaspoon kosher salt

1 6-ounce carton plain low-fat or fat-free yogurt

⅓ cup finely chopped, seeded cucumber

2 tablespoons chopped fresh mint

⅛ teaspoon kosher salt

⅛ teaspoon freshly ground black pepper

Nutrition facts per serving: 366 cal., 14 g total fat (5 g sat. fat), 152 mg chol., 270 mg sodium, 6 g carbo., 1 g fiber, 51 g pro.
Exchanges: ½ Vegetable, 7 Very Lean Meat, 2½ Fat

*Note: Because hot chile peppers contain oils that can burn your skin and eyes, wear rubber or plastic gloves when working with them. If your bare hands do touch the chile peppers, wash your hands well with soap and water.

**Note: If you don't have a small food processor, finely chop chile peppers, cilantro, and green onions. In a small bowl combine chopped chile peppers, cilantro, green onions, lemon juice, olive oil, and ⅛ teaspoon kosher salt.

For Wave 1, serve with a mixed green salad and cooked bulgur. For Waves 2 and 3, serve with a mixed green salad, cooked bulgur, and fresh grapes.

Source: Chef Toni, Windsor Vineyards

Wine Pairing: Zinfandel

1. Preheat broiler. Trim fat from chops; set aside. In a small food processor°° combine the chile peppers, cilantro, green onions, lemon juice, olive oil, and ⅛ teaspoon kosher salt. Cover and process until finely chopped. Using the back of a small spoon or a metal spatula, spread the chile pepper mixture over both sides of the chops.

2. Place chops on the unheated rack of a broiler pan. Broil 3 to 4 inches from the heat for 10 to 15 minutes or until medium doneness (160°F), turning once halfway through broiling.

3. Meanwhile, in a small bowl combine yogurt, cucumber, mint, ⅛ teaspoon kosher salt, and the black pepper. Serve with lamb.

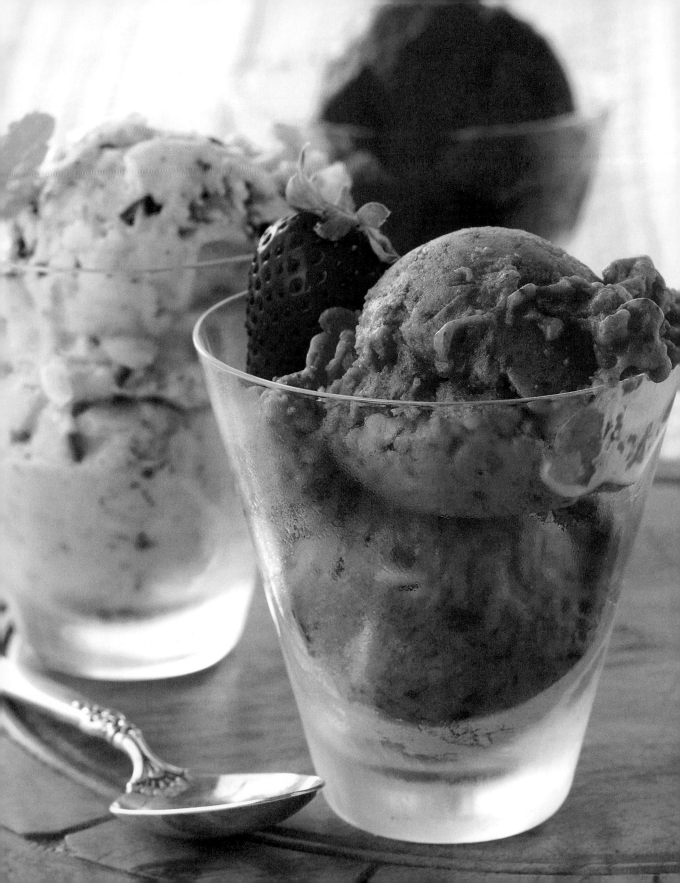

FROZEN FRUIT "SORBET"

Chef Toni Sakaguchi suggests using fresh, ripe fruit for these recipes. The taste of the ripe fruit will be so sweet that you won't miss the sugar in this creamy, light dessert.

Prep: 10 minutes **Freeze:** 1½ hours **Makes:** 4 (about ½-cup) servings

2 medium bananas

1 cup sliced strawberries

2 tablespoons water

1 tablespoon lemon juice

Fresh strawberries (optional)

1. Peel bananas and cut into 1-inch pieces. Place banana slices and strawberries in a waxed-paper-lined 15×10×1-inch baking pan. Cover and freeze for 1½ to 2 hours or until completely frozen. In a food processor combine frozen fruit, the water, and lemon juice. Cover and process until smooth. If desired, garnish with fresh strawberries.

Per serving: 65 cal., 0 g total fat (0 g sat. fat), 0 mg chol., 1 mg sodium, 17 g carbo., 2 g fiber, 1 g pro.
Exchanges: 1 Fruit

Banana-Chocolate "Sorbet": Peel 3 medium bananas and cut into 1-inch pieces. Place banana slices in a waxed-paper-lined 15×10×1-inch baking pan. Cover and freeze for 1½ to 2 hours or until completely frozen. In a food processor combine frozen bananas, 2 tablespoons water, and 1 tablespoon bittersweet chocolate pieces. Cover and process until nearly smooth (will still have small bits of hard chocolate). If desired, garnish with fresh mint leaves.

Nutrition facts per serving: 91 cal., 1 g total fat (0 g sat. fat), 0 mg chol., 1 mg sodium, 22 g carbo., 3 g fiber, 1 g pro.
Exchanges: 1 Fruit, ½ Other Carbo.

Peach-Raspberry "Sorbet": Place 2 cups peach slices and 1 cup raspberries in a waxed-paper-lined 15×10×1-inch baking pan. Cover with waxed paper and freeze about 45 minutes or until partially frozen. In a food processor combine fruit, 1 tablespoon honey, and 1 tablespoon lemon juice. Cover and process until smooth. If desired, garnish with fresh raspberries.

Nutrition facts per serving: 69 cal., 0 g total fat (0 g sat. fat), 0 mg chol., 1 mg sodium, 18 g carbo., 4 g fiber, 1 g pro.
Exchanges: 1 Fruit

Source: Toni Sakaguchi, Chef Instructor at The Culinary Institute of America
In honor of Chef Catherine Brandel

INDEX

Boldfaced page references indicate photographs.

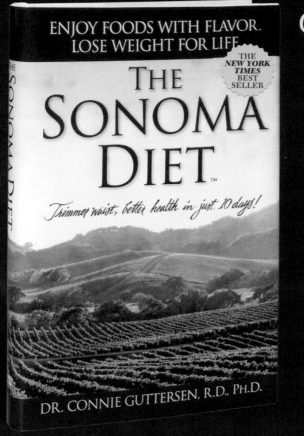